AF412727

BRUCE H. THIERS, MD, Consulting Editor

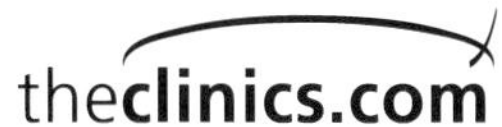

DERMATOLOGIC CLINICS

Drug Actions, Reactions, and Interactions

JAMES Q. DEL ROSSO, DO, FAOCD

Guest Editor

April 2007 • Volume 25 • Number 2

SAUNDERS

An Imprint of Elsevier, Inc.
PHILADELPHIA   LONDON   TORONTO   MONTREAL   SYDNEY   TOKYO

W.B. SAUNDERS COMPANY
A Division of Elsevier Inc.

Elsevier Inc. • 1600 John F. Kennedy Blvd., Suite 1800 • Philadelphia, Pennsylvania 19103-2899

http://www.theclinics.com

DERMATOLOGIC CLINICS
April 2007
Editor: Alexandra Gavenda

Volume 25, Number 2
ISSN 0733-8635
ISBN 1-4160-4305-5
978-1-4160-4305-8

The ideas and opinions expressed in *Dermatologic Clinics* do not necessarily reflect those of the Publisher. The Publisher does not assume any responsibility for any injury and/or damage to persons or property arising out of or related to any use of the material contained in this periodical. The reader is advised to check the appropriate medical literature and the product information currently provided by the manufacturer of each drug to be administered to verify the dosage, the method and duration of administration, or contraindications. It is the responsibility of the treating physician or other health care professional, relying on independent experience and knowledge of the patient, to determine drug dosages and the best treatment for the patient. Mention of any product in this issue should not be construed as endorsement by the contributors, editors, or the Publisher of the product or manufacturers' claims.

Dermatologic Clinics (ISSN 0733-8635) is published quarterly by Elsevier Inc., 360 Park Avenue South, New York, NY 10010-1710. Months of publication are January, April, July, and October. Business and editorial offices: 1600 John F. Kennedy Blvd., Suite 1800, Philadelphia, PA 19103-2899. Customer service office: 6277 Sea Harbor Drive, Orlando, FL 32887-4800. Periodicals postage paid at New York, NY, and additional mailing offices. Subscription prices are USD 231 per year for US individuals, USD 356 per year for US institutions, USD 270 per year for Canadian individuals, USD 416 per year for Canadian institutions, USD 297 per year for international individuals, USD 416 per year for international institutions, USD 110 per year for US students, USD 149 per year for Canadian students, and USD 149 per year for international students. International air speed delivery is included in all *Clinics* subscription prices. All prices are subject to change without notice. POSTMASTER: Send address changes to *Dermatologic Clinics*, Elsevier Periodicals Customer Service, 6277 Sea Harbor Drive, Orlando, FL 32887-4800. **Customer Service: 1-800-654-2452 (US). From outside of the US, call 1-407-345-4000. E-mail: hhspcs@harcourt.com.**

Reprints. For copies of 100 or more, of articles in this publication, please contact the Commercial Reprints Department, Elsevier Inc., 360 Park Avenue South, New York, New York 10010-1710. Tel.: (212) 633-3813; Fax: (212) 462-1935; Email: repritns@elsevier.com.

The *Dermatologic Clinics* is covered in *Index Medicus, Current Contents/Clinical Medicine, Excerpta Medica, Chemical Abstracts,* and *ISI/BIOMED.*

Printed in the United States of America.

GUEST EDITOR

JAMES Q. DEL ROSSO, DO, FAOCD, Dermatology Residency Director, Valley Hospital Medical Center, Las Vegas, Nevada

CONTRIBUTORS

JOERG ALBRECHT, MD, Department of Medicine, Division of Dermatology, John Stroger Jr Hospital of Cook County, Chicago, Illinois

NEIL BHATIA, MD, Assistant Clinical Professor, University of Wisconsin Medical School, Milwaukee, Wisconsin

JEFFREY P. CALLEN, MD, Professor of Medicine (Dermatology) and Chief, Division of Dermatology, University of Louisville School of Medicine, Louisville, Kentucky

WILLIAM L. CAMP, MD, MPH, Department of Medicine, University of Alabama at Birmingham, Birmingham, Alabama

SHARI B. CLARKE, MD, Department of Dermatology, The Pennsylvania State University College of Medicine, Hershey, Pennsylvania

JAMES Q. DEL ROSSO, DO, FAOCD, Dermatology Residency Director, Valley Hospital Medical Center, Las Vegas, Nevada

ALPESH DESAI, DO, Director, Heights Dermatology and Aesthetic Center, Houston, Texas; Professor of Dermatology, Western University of Health Sciences, Pomona, California

BONI E. ELEWSKI, MD, Department of Dermatology, University of Alabama at Birmingham, Birmingham, Alabama

DIRK M. ELSTON, MD, Director, Department of Dermatology; and Department of Pathology, Geisinger Medical Center, Danville, Pennsylvania

LAUREN ANN FINE, MD, Department of Medicine, Division of Dermatology, John Stroger Jr Hospital of Cook County, Chicago, Illinois

ROSALYN E. GEORGE, MD, Department of Dermatology, The Pennsylvania State University College of Medicine, Hershey, Pennsylvania

MATILDE IORIZZO, MD, Department of Dermatology, University of Bologna, Bologna, Italy

FRANCISCA KARTONO, BS, Western University of Health Sciences, Pomona, California

SANDRA R. KNOWLES, BScPhm, Lecturer, Faculty of Pharmacy, University of Toronto; and Sunnybrook Health Sciences Centre, Drug Safety Clinic, Toronto, Ontario, Canada

MARK LEBWOHL, MD, Department of Dermatology, Mount Sinai Medical Center, New York, New York

JAMES J. LEYDEN, MD, Emeritus Professor of Dermatology, University of Pennsylvania, Philadelphia, Pennsylvania

AMANDA M. NELSON, PhD, The Jake Gittlen Cancer Research Foundation, The Pennsylvania State University College of Medicine, Hershey, Pennsylvania

MASSIMILIANO PAZZAGLIA, MD, Department of Dermatology, University of Bologna, Bologna, Italy

WARREN PIETTE, MD, Chair, Department of Medicine, Division of Dermatology, John Stroger Jr Hospital of Cook County; and Professor, Department of Dermatology, Rush Medical Center, Chicago, Illinois

BIANCA MARIA PIRACCINI, MD, PhD, Department of Dermatology, University of Bologna, Bologna, Italy

KATHLEEN REMLINGER, MD, Associate Professor of Dermatology, Rush-Presbyterian-St. Luke's Medical Center, Chicago, Illinois

NEIL H. SHEAR, MD, FRCPC, FACP, Helen and Paul Phelan Professor and Chief of Dermatology, Faculty of Medicine, University of Toronto; and Sunnybrook Health Sciences Centre, Drug Safety Clinic, Toronto, Ontario, Canada

DIANE M. THIBOUTOT, MD, Department of Dermatology; and The Jake Gittlen Research Foundation, The Pennsylvania State University College of Medicine, Hershey, Pennsylvania

ANTONELLA TOSTI, MD, Department of Dermatology, University of Bologna, Bologna, Italy

GUY WEBSTER, MD, PhD, Department of Dermatology, Jefferson Medical College, Philadelphia, Pennsylvania

STEPHEN E. WOLVERTON, MD, Professor of Clinical Dermatology and Vice-Chair of Clinical Affairs, Indiana University Medical Center, Department of Dermatology, Indianapolis, Indiana

JOSHUA A. ZEICHNER, MD, Department of Dermatology, Mount Sinai Medical Center, New York, New York

ALEXANDRA Y. ZHANG, MD, Department of Dermatology, University of Alabama at Birmingham, Birmingham, Alabama

CONTENTS

armamentarium. Drugs of greatest interest concerning hepatic toxicity include methotrexate, azathioprine, dapsone, and acitretin. Somewhat overlapping are drugs that have important hematologic toxicities, including methotrexate, azathioprine, dapsone, sulfonamides, cyclophosphamide, and chlorambucil. Laboratory tests most commonly used include (1) hepatic monitoring: transaminases (AST/SGOT and ALT/SGPT) and the ultrasound-guided liver biopsy, and (2) hematologic monitoring: CBC with diff and platelets along with occasional use of the reticulocyte count. Important principles and specific guidelines for monitoring by drug group are highlighted.

Potential Complications Associated with the Use of Biologic Agents for Psoriasis

Joshua A. Zeichner and Mark Lebwohl

The biologic agents are effective drugs to treat psoriasis. They provide physicians with additional options for patients who cannot tolerate traditional therapies or for whom traditional therapies are not sufficient. While these new TNF-α inhibitors and anti–T-cell agents have potential complications, they are generally safe with proper monitoring. Both physicians and patients should be aware of the risks involved with each medicine so that the correct drug is chosen to suit each patient.

Drug Reactions Affecting the Nail Unit: Diagnosis and Management

Bianca Maria Piraccini and Matilde Iorizzo

Several drugs may be responsible for the development of nail abnormalities, but only a few classes are consistently associated with nail symptoms. Drug-induced nail abnormalities result from toxicity to the matrix, the nail bed, the periungual tissues, or the digit blood vessels. Pharmacologic agents that most frequently produce nail abnormalities include retinoids, indinavir, and cancer chemotherapeutic agents.

Drug Reactions Affecting Hair: Diagnosis

Antonella Tosti and Massimiliano Pazzaglia

Drugs may cause hair loss, stimulate hair growth, or induce changes in the hair shape and color. Drug-induced hair loss is, in most cases, a consequence of a toxic effect of the drug on the hair matrix. Although a large number of drugs have been occasionally reported to produce hair loss, the relationship between drug intake and hair loss has been proven only for a few agents. Type of hair loss (telogen effluvium, anagen effluvium, or both) depends on the drug, its dosage, and patient's susceptibility. Drug-induced hair loss is usually reversible.

Drug-Associated Lymphoma and Pseudolymphoma: Recognition and Management

Joerg Albrecht, Lauren Ann Fine, and Warren Piette

This article discusses ways to recognize and manage lymphomas and pseudolymphomas associated with drug exposure. Over the last 30 years, the classification of pseudolymphomas and lymphomas has undergone significant change, especially following the application of sophisticated immunostaining and gene rearrangement analysis. The term cutaneous pseudolymphomas (CPL) is a nonspecific term for a heterogeneous group of benign reactive T- or B-cell lymphoproliferative processes that simulate cutaneous lymphomas clinically or histologically. While pseudolymphomas are relatively rare diseases, their clinical and histological heterogeneity has led to multiple systems of categorization based on immunological factors, causative agents, presentation, and clinical course.

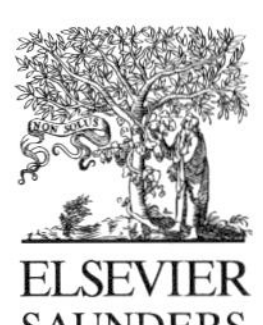

ELSEVIER
SAUNDERS

Dermatol Clin 25 (2007) xi–xii

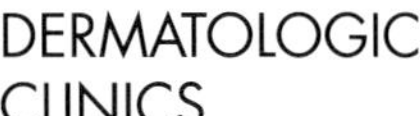

DERMATOLOGIC
CLINICS

Preface

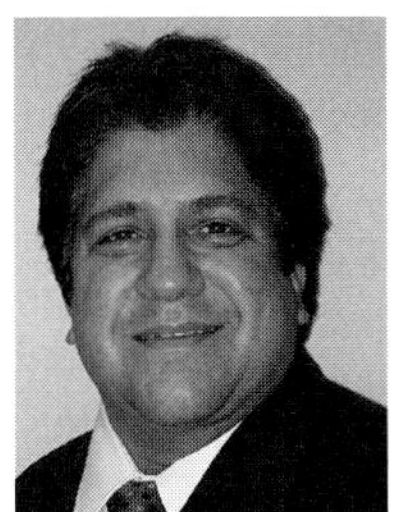

James Q. Del Rosso, DO, FAOCD
Guest Editor

It is with great pleasure and pride that I bring to you this issue of the *Dermatologic Clinics*. When I was invited by Dr. Bruce Thiers to develop and edit the April 2007 issue covering drug actions, reactions, and interactions, I accepted without hesitation. The opportunity to select topics of importance to dermatologists, especially clinicians working "in the trenches," has proven to be one of the high points of my career in dermatology.

I have tried to pull together a collection of important topics covered by leaders in their field who are capable of providing up-to-date information and who can translate their knowledge to the clinician. The subjects that are covered in this issue are varied and reflect my attempt to include clinically relevant topics, some of which are not commonly presented in a comprehensive manner within a single reference.

The drug actions component of this issue focuses on timely topics such as antibiotic resistance, including a special focus on methicillin-resistant *Staphylococcus aureus*, topical immunomodulator therapies, pharmacologic modulation of sebaceous gland activity, systemic retinoid therapy, antifungal agents, and anti-inflammatory effects of antibiotic drugs. The term *antibiotic* is commonly used to classify these drugs within a recognizable category; however, it more accurately describes an activity or effect. Many agents capable of exhibiting antibiotic activity (eg, tetracyclines), exhibit many biologic effects unrelated to their antibiotic capabilities.

The drug reactions and interactions segment covers more recently recognized drug reactions, adverse reactions associated with biologic agents, drug-associated pseudolymphoma, drug reactions affecting hair and nails, recognition and monitoring of potential hepatotoxic and hematologic reactions, and a thorough discussion of more severe cutaneous drug eruptions. The reviews of systemic retinoids and antifungal agents include discussions on adverse effects and interactions.

My hope is that this issue remains close at hand as an important reference in day-to-day dermatology practice. I am very thankful to all of the authors for the time and effort they contributed. I owe much gratitude to several dermatologists who have positively influenced my career and sustained my interest in dermatology—including my first

derm.theclinics.com

mentor, Dr. Robert Verona, and my residency director, Dr. David Horowitz. I would be remiss if I did not recognize my parents, Quinten and Antoinette Del Rosso, who made sure I fully understood that mediocrity is not acceptable, and my sister, Marilyn Lanza, who taught me that tackling any project without passion is a waste of time. Finally, and of utmost importance, I want to thank the love of my life, my wife Karyn, for her perpetual patience and support as I dedicate so much of my time and energy to educational endeavors in dermatology, such as this April 2007 issue of the *Dermatologic Clinics*.

James Q. Del Rosso, DO, FAOCD
Valley Hospital Medical Center
620 Shadow Lane
Las Vegas, NV 89106, USA

E-mail address: jqdelrosso@yahoo.com

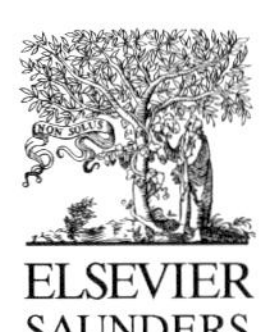

Dermatol Clin 25 (2007) 127–132

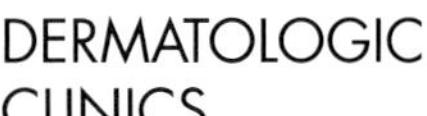

Status Report on Antibiotic Resistance: Implications for the Dermatologist

James Q. Del Rosso, DO, FAOCD[a],*, James J. Leyden, MD[b]

[a]*Valley Hospital Medical Center, PMB-531, 3230 E. Flamingo Road #8, Las Vegas, NV 89121, USA*
[b]*University of Pennsylvania, 3451 Walnut Street, Philadelphia, PA 19104, USA*

The use of antibiotics, both oral and topical, is common in dermatologic practice, including the use for treatment of bacterial infections and inflammatory dermatoses such as acne vulgaris, rosacea, perioral dermatitis, and some immunobullous diseases [1]. Based on data from 2003, dermatologists accounted for 8.8 million oral antibiotic prescriptions, representing 19.6% of all prescriptions written by dermatologists [2]. During this same annual time period, tetracyclines accounted for 65% of oral antibiotics prescribed by dermatologists, followed by cephalosporins (10%) and erythromycin (8%). The remaining 17% was distributed among penicillin derivatives, quinolones, other macrolides, and trimethoprim-sulfamethoxazole. Among the oral tetracycline agents alone, 51.4% of prescriptions were for minocycline, 30.6% for doxycycline, and 18% for tetracycline.

In the United States and worldwide, public awareness of the progressive rise in antibiotic resistance has increased among public health officials, the medical community, and the lay public [3–7]. In response to educational initiatives designed to decrease overall antibiotic use in the United Kingdom, oral antibiotic prescribing by general practitioners for acne vulgaris decreased by 33% from 1996 to 2000 [6]. Over the same 5-year time period, prescribing of systemic antibiotics by pediatricians declined in the United States by 25% and 16% in children aged 3 to less than 6 years and 6 to less than 18 years, respectively [8]. In 2004, the US Food and Drug Administration (FDA) mandated official labeling changes in

product monographs for systemic antibiotics emphasizing the need for cautious and directed prescribing [9].

How does antibiotic resistance develop?

With a "stockpile of more than 100 drugs" available since the 1940s, antibiotic use in medicine is widespread [5]. From 1954 to 1998, antibiotic production in the United States increased from 2 million to over 50 million pounds, a rise reflective of overall use including medicinal and agricultural. Bacteria become resistant to antibiotics through a variety of genetic and biologic mechanisms [5,10]. A major factor related to antibiotic resistance among bacteria is selection pressure. In the absence of antibiotic exposure, commensal and transient bacterial flora, including opportunistic pathogens, live in a competitive environment, limiting the proliferation of potential pathogens [5,10]. Upon antibiotic exposure, especially with chronic or frequent use, the population of susceptible bacterial strains is significantly reduced, leaving behind resistant organisms that can then proliferate owing to reduced competition. The remaining resistant organisms can transfer their resistance genes to other species, amplifying antibiotic resistance patterns [5].

Genetic variability among bacteria is related to three major mechanisms that produce changes correlated with the production of resistance genes [5,11]. Microevolutionary change results from point nucleotide mutations that may change antibiotic target sites or alter production of antibiotic-inactivating enzymes [11]. An example of the latter includes point mutations of preexisting beta-lactamase genes, ultimately producing multiple

* Corresponding author.
E-mail address: jqdelrosso@yahoo.com
(J.Q. Del Rosso).

new extended-spectrum beta-lactamase enzymes [10–12]. Macroevolutionary change creates major alterations in large DNA segments, which may include transposition of large sequences between locations on bacterial chromosomes or plasmids [10,11]. Plasmids are extrachromosomal mobile DNA elements that may spread specific antibiotic resistance genes within and between bacterial species [11,13,14]. Alterations of the bacterial genome are commonly produced as major genetic components referred to as transposons and insertion sequences and are capable of independent movement from the bacterial genome. A third method of transfer of antibiotic resistance among bacteria occurs when organisms acquire foreign DNA via mobile genetic elements such as plasmids or bacteriophages [11]. Recognition of the ability of bacteria of different genera and species to transfer genetic determinants of antibiotic resistance is increasing as exemplified by apparent transfer of beta-lactam and aminoglycoside resistance from staphylococci to enterococci [11,15–17]. Tables 1 and 2 provide a detailed outline of mechanisms involved in the development of antibiotic resistance among bacteria. Table 3 lists individual antibiotics and related mechanisms of antibiotic resistance.

Antibiotic resistance and dermatologic practice

The common use of systemic antibiotic therapy in dermatology warrants a closer look at how prescribing patterns impact on the development of antibiotic resistant bacteria and outcomes in clinical practice. Considerations include use for common inflammatory disorders such as acne vulgaris, their impact on commensal and transient flora, and changes in resistance patterns among pathogens causing common skin and soft tissue infections [4,6,7].

Acne vulgaris

The role of *Propionibacterium acnes* in the pathogenesis of acne is well established [18]. Antibiotic-resistant *P acnes* prevalence rates increased from 20% to 62% from 1978 to 1996 based on an analysis of global data, and European analyses report tetracycline-resistant and erythromycin-resistant *P acnes* strains in up to 20% and 50% of patients, respectively [4,19,20]. In the United States, minocycline produces the greatest log reduction of *P acnes* and the lowest incidence of *P acnes* resistance [21,22]. Although several factors influence the response to acne treatment, antibiotic-resistant strains of *P acnes* have been correlated in some cases with reduced therapeutic benefit [6,18]. Benzoyl peroxide has been shown to decrease emergence of antibiotic-resistant *P acnes* organisms and to reduce the proliferation of antibiotic-resistant *P acnes* strains present before the initiation of antibiotic therapy [23].

Impact on commensal and transient flora

When an oral antibiotic is ingested, the microbial ecosystem of the host is altered as commensal and transient skin and mucosal flora undergo antibiotic exposure [5]. The use of antibiotics commonly prescribed in dermatology, such as

Table 1
Mechanisms of genetic variability among bacteria related to transfer of antibiotic resistance

Mechanism	Implications
Plasmids	Extrachromosomal double-stranded DNA elements/variable size
	Influence multiple functions (resistance, virulence, metabolism)
	Plasmid DNA transferable between bacterial species
	Conjugate plasmids may transfer among species, producing resistance in previously sensitive strains
Transferable genetic elements	Includes transposons and insertion sequences (mobile elements)
	May translocate within bacterial chromosome or between chromosome and plasmid or bacteriophage
	Conjugate transposons may transpose directly from chromosome of one bacteria to another
Integration elements	Represent closely linked genetic material consecutively sequenced along bacterial chromosome or plasmid forming integrated units (integrons)
	Provide location for insertion of foreign DNA resistance genes

Data from Refs. [11–17].

Table 2
Mechanisms of antibiotic resistance among bacteria

Mechanism	Implications
Enzymatic inactivation	Resistance genes inducing production of enzymes that inactivate or modify specific antibiotics
	Examples include beta-lactamases, erythromycin esterase, and aminoglycoside resistance-modifying enzymes
Alteration of outer membrane permeability	Hydrophilic antibiotics pass through arranged protein channels (porins)
	Mutation-induced loss of specific porins and other outer membrane proteins may confer antibiotic resistance
Antibiotic efflux	Reduced antibiotic uptake by bacteria due to membrane protein produced by a resistance determinant
	Increased antibiotic efflux across cell membrane
	Examples include decreased uptake and efflux of tetracyclines, resistance of some staphylococci and streptococci to macrolides and azalides, and beta-lactamase resistance in *Pseudomonas aeruginosa*
Alteration of ribosomal target sites	Enzymatic change of ribosomal binding sites inhibits antibiotic binding
	Resistance examples include tetracyclines, macrolides, and lincosamides
Alteration of cell wall targets	Modification of terminal foci on peptidoglycan precursors prevents antibiotic binding
	Resistance includes glycopeptide antibiotics such as vancomycin and teicoplanin
Alteration of target enzymes	Alteration of target proteins (eg, penicillin-binding proteins) prevents beta-lactam antibiotic binding in the cytoplasmic membrane, resulting in antibiotic resistance
	Mutations in loci on DNA-gyrase induce quinolone resistance

Data from Refs. [10,11,36].

tetracyclines and erythromycin, has been associated with the development of resistant strains of *P acnes* and coagulase-negative staphylococci, leading to a proliferation of resistant bacteria in the skin and gastrointestinal tract of treated patients and their close family contacts [4,6,24–27]. Antibiotic therapy administered over a period of at least 3 months for acne vulgaris has been shown

Table 3
Antibiotics and related resistance mechanisms

Drug category	Mechanisms of antibiotic resistance
Tetracyclines	Alteration of ribosomal binding target
	Active drug efflux/reduced drug uptake
Macrolides/lincosamides	Alteration of ribosomal binding target
	Limited drug permeability/reduced drug uptake
	Active drug efflux
	Enzymatic drug inactivation
Beta-lactams	Altered membrane-binding proteins
	Limited drug permeability/reduced drug uptake
	Enzymatic drug inactivation
Quinolones	Alteration of enzyme target (DNA-gyrase)
	Limited drug permeability/reduced drug uptake
	Active drug efflux

Data from Opal SM, Mayer KH, Medeiros AA. Mechanisms of bacterial antibiotic resistance. In: Mandell GL, Bennett JE, Dolin R, editors. Principles and practice of infectious disease. 5th edition. Philadelphia: Churchill-Livingston; 2000. p. 236–51; and Eliopoulos GM. Mechanisms of bacterial resistance to antimicrobial drugs. In: Gorbach SL, Bartlett JG, Blacklow NR, editors. Infectious diseases. 2nd edition. Philadelphia: WB Saunders; 1998. p. 319–30.

to increase oropharyngeal colonization of *Streptococcus pyogenes*, with a higher rate of antibiotic resistance for this organism when compared with the rate in an untreated group of patients with acne (control group) [28]. In this study, patients who had acne when treated with antibiotic therapy exhibited a 33% positive culture rate for *S pyogenes* from the oropharynx compared with a 10% rate in controls. Eighty-five percent of the *S pyogenes* organisms cultured from the group treated with antibiotics were resistant to at least one tetracycline agent compared with 20% of those cultured from the untreated group. Concern has been expressed that chronic antibiotic exposure for disorders such as acne vulgaris may evoke multiple resistance mechanisms, producing a readily available pool of mobile resistance genes that may be transferred among multiple bacterial strains, including staphylococci [6,29]. As a result, some authorities have suggested that the use of long-term antibiotic therapy for acne vulgaris be reconsidered, although a consensus and definitive guidelines have not been established [4,6,29,30]. Further research is needed to more clearly define the clinical implications of prolonged antibiotic administration for disorders such as acne vulgaris and rosacea.

Implications in skin and soft tissue infections

Bacterial skin and soft tissue infections are commonly encountered in community practice and in institutional settings. As many as 17% of skin-related complaints presenting in pediatric clinics are due to bacterial infection [7,31].

Folliculitis, cellulitis, and impetigo caused by gram-positive cocci (eg, *Staphylococcus aureus, S*

pyogenes) are the most common bacterial skin infections encountered in the ambulatory setting in general and dermatology practice [7]. Owing to antibiotic exposure over time, resistance patterns in cutaneous bacterial pathogens have emerged that are of potential clinical significance (Table 4) [7,32–34]. Despite the availability of several newer antibiotics, most uncomplicated skin and soft tissue infections encountered in ambulatory practice respond favorably to conventional agents such as cephalexin, cefdinir, and amoxicillin-clavulanate [7]. Newer agents such as linezolid and several fluoroquinolones (eg, gatifloxacin, avlofloxacin) have not been shown to be more effective than conventional agents for infections caused by methicillin-sensitive *S aureus* or *S pyogenes*, and these newer agents are best withheld "unless the causative pathogen mandates their use" [7]. Community-acquired methicillin-resistant *S aureus* (CAMRSA) continues to increase in prevalence across the United States, exhibiting antibiotic susceptibility patterns and genetic resistance elements that differ from hospital-acquired resistant strains (HAMRSA) [35]. CAMRSA strains are often susceptible to trimethoprim-sulfamethoxazole, minocycline, or doxycycline, with durations of therapy ranging from at least 10 to 21 days required in uncomplicated cases [35]. Although quinolones are often reported to be active in vitro against CAMRSA, rapid develop of *S aureus* resistance to quinolones is common [35].

Antibiotic cross-resistance

When members of a given structural antibiotic class bind to the same bacterial target sites,

Table 4
Resistance patterns of clinically significant dermatologic bacterial isolates

Pathogen/resistance pattern	Reported rates of resistance
Methicillin-resistant *S aureus*	21% (Japan, 2000)
	13% (United Kingdom, 2000)
	31% (Latin America, 1998)
Macrolide-resistant *S aureus*	10%–20% (United States, 2002)
	28% (Israel, 1990)
	39% (Japan, 2000)
	30% (United Kingdom, 2000)
Macrolide-resistant *S pyogenes*	18% (United Kingdom, 2000)
	3%–7.7% (United States, 1999)
Mupirocin-resistant *S aureus*	3% (MRSA strains; United States, 2003)
	0.3%–0.4% (non-MRSA strains; United States, 2003)
	20% (New Zealand, 2003)
	10% (United Kingdom burn units, 2003)
	11% (chronic therapy up to 4 years)

Data from Refs. [7,32–34].

demonstrate similar pharmacokinetic properties, and are susceptible to degradation by the same enzymes, antibiotic cross-resistance is likely [36]. Antibiotic cross-resistance is not always predictable based on susceptibility testing. In some cases, antibiotics in the same chemical class may appear to exhibit cross-resistance with specific organisms in vitro; however, clinical disease may respond owing to differences in drug concentration at the target site [6]. Differences in potency among drugs in the same chemical category may also have a role. For example, bacterial strains resistant to cephalexin, including *S aureus*, are frequently susceptible in vitro to cefdinir; 84% of cephalexin-resistant isolates have been reported to be susceptible to cefdinir [37].

Guidelines for reduction of antibiotic resistance

Increasing concerns regarding antibiotic resistance should encourage clinicians to examine their antibiotic prescribing patterns without jeopardizing the treatment of patients in need of therapy. Decisions must be weighed based on factors specific to each individual case. In acne vulgaris, systemic antibiotic use is based on the response to previous therapies and disease severity. Although it has been suggested that oral antibiotic therapy for acne be restricted to 6 months or less of use, this approach is not always practical; some patients experience rapid rebound after discontinuation, despite use of a topical regimen [6].

It is prudent to limit the duration of oral antibiotic use whenever possible and to control acne with a rational topical program. Antibiotics should not be used as monotherapy for acne vulgaris [6]. In rosacea, systemic antibiotic therapy may be minimized or avoided with the use of an anti-inflammatory dose of doxycycline. This approach depends on anti-inflammatory and anticollagenolytic effects and is devoid of antibiotic activity, even with long-term use [38]. The use of an anti-inflammatory dose of doxycycline that is devoid of antibiotic activity may also be of benefit in the treatment of acne vulgaris; however, the response to treatment may be slower [39].

With regard to the treatment of uncomplicated bacterial infections commonly encountered in ambulatory dermatology practice, clinical judgment in combination with rational antibiotic selection is usually sufficient. In most cases, conventional agents (eg, cefdinir, amoxicillin-clavulanate) prove to be effective. Culture and sensitivity may assist in identifying pathogens or antibiotic susceptibility patterns (eg, CAMRSA) that warrant a change in antibiotic therapy. The use of topical mupirocin should be limited to short courses, preferably in confirmed cases of *S aureus* infection, because chronic mupirocin application has been associated with a significant increase in resistant *S aureus* isolates [7,34].

References

[1] Del Rosso JQ. Systemic therapy for rosacea: focus on oral antibiotic therapy and safety. Cutis 2000; 66(Suppl):7–13.

[2] Del Rosso JQ, Elston DM, Hirschmann J, et al. Summary report from the Scientific Panel on antibiotic use in dermatology: usage patterns, management challenges recommendations (poster presentation). American Academy of Dermatology Summer Meeting, San Diego, CA, July 26–30, 2006.

[3] Kunin CM. Resistance to antimicrobial drugs—a worldwide calamity. Ann Intern Med 1993;118: 557–61.

[4] Espersen F. Resistance to antibiotics used in dermatological practice. Br J Dermatol 1998;139:4–8.

[5] Levy SB. The challenge of antibiotic resistance. Sci Am 1998;278:46–53.

[6] Eady AH, Cove JH, Layton AM. Is antibiotic resistance in cutaneous propionibacteria clinically relevant? Implications of resistance for acne patients and prescribers. Am J Clin Dermatol 2003;12: 813–31.

[7] Guay DRP. Treatment of bacterial skin and skin structure infections. Expert Opin Pharmacother 2003;4:1259–75.

[8] Finkelstein JA, Stille C, Nordin J, et al. Reduction in antibiotic use among US children 1996–2000. Pediatrics 2003;139:467–71.

[9] FDA to require warning labels on antibiotics. Health Care Business Daily. February 6, 2003.

[10] Gold HS, Moellering RC Jr. Antimicrobial drug resistance. N Engl J Med 1996;335:1445–53.

[11] Opal SM, Mayer KH, Medeiros AA. Mechanisms of bacterial antibiotic resistance. In: Mandell GL, Bennett JE, Dolin R, editors. Principles and practice of infectious disease. 5th edition. Philadelphia: Churchill-Livingstone; 2000. p. 236–51.

[12] Medeiros AA. Evolution and dissemination of beta-lactamase accelerated by generations of beta-lactam antibiotics. Clin Infect Dis 1997;24:S19–45.

[13] Timmis KN, Gonzalez-Carrero MI, Sekizaki T, et al. Biological activities specified by antibiotic resistance plasmids. J Antimicrob Chemother 1986; 18(Suppl C):1–12.

[14] O'Brien T, Pla MP, Mayer KH, et al. Intercontinental spread of a new antibiotic resistance gene on an epidemic plasmid. Science 1985;230:87–8.

[15] Brisson-Noel A, Arthur M, Courvalin P. Evidence for natural gene transfer from gram-positive cocci to *Escherichia coli*. J Bacteriol 1988;170:1739–45.

[16] Courvalin P, Carlier C, Collatz E. Plasmid-mediated resistance to aminocyclitol antibiotics in group D streptococci. J Bacteriol 1980;143:541–51.

[17] Zscheck KK, Hull R, Murray BE, et al. Restriction mapping and hybridization studies of a beta-lactamase-encoding fragment from *Streptococcus (Enterococcus) faecalis*. Antimicrob Agents Chemother 1988;32:768–9.

[18] Leyden JJ. The evolving role of *Propionibacterium acnes* in acne. Semin Cutan Med Surg 2001;20: 139–43.

[19] Cooper AJ. Systematic review of *Propionibacterium acnes* resistance to systemic antibiotics. Med J Aust 1998;169:259–61.

[20] Ross JI, Snelling AM, Carnegie E, et al. Antibiotic resistant acne: lessons from Europe. Br J Dermatol 2003;148:467–78.

[21] Kligman A. Comparison of topical benzoyl peroxide gel, oral minocycline, oral doxycycline and a combination for suppression of *P acnes* in acne patients. J Dermatolog Treat 1998;9:187–91.

[22] Ross JI, Snelling AM, Eady EA, et al. Phenotypic and genotypic characterization of antibiotic-resistant *Propionibacterium acnes* isolated from acne patients attending dermatology clinics in Europe, the USA, Japan and Australia. Br J Dermatol 2001; 144:339–46.

[23] Eady EA, Bojar RA, Jones CE, et al. The effects of acne treatment with a combination of benzoyl peroxide and erythromycin on skin carriage of erythromycin-resistant propionibacteria. Br J Dermatol 1996;134:107–13.

[24] Leyden JJ, McGinley KJ, Cavalieri S, et al. *Propionibacterium acnes* resistance to antibiotics in acne patients. J Am Acad Dermatol 1983;8:41–5.

[25] Miller YW, Eady EA, Lacey RW, et al. Sequential antibiotic therapy for acne promotes the carriage of resistant staphylococci on the skin of contacts. J Antimicrob Chemother 1996;38:829–37.

[26] Marples RR, Kligman AM. Ecological effect of oral antibiotics on the microflora of human skin. Arch Dermatol 1971;103:148–53.

[27] Adams SJ, Cunliffe WJ, Cooke EM. Long-term antibiotic therapy for acne vulgaris: effects on the bowel flora of patients and their relatives. J Invest Dermatol 1985;85:35–7.

[28] Levy RM, Huang EY, Roling D, et al. Effect of antibiotics on the oropharyngeal flora in patients with acne. Arch Dermatol 2003;139:467–71.

[29] Eady EA. Bacterial resistance in acne. Dermatology 1998;196:59–66.

[30] Cheesbrough MJ. Antibiotics should not be first treatment for acne [letter]. BMJ 1999;318:669.

[31] Hayden GF. Skin diseases encountered in a pediatric clinic: a one-year prospective study. Am J Dis Child 1985;139:36–8.

[32] Finerty EF, Polan DW Jr. Changing antibiotic sensitivities of bacterial skin diseases: office practices. Cutis 1979;23:227–30.

[33] Nishijima S, Kurakowa I. Antimicrobial resistance of *Staphylococcus aureus* isolated from skin infections. Int J Antimicrob Agents 2002;19:241–3.

[34] Moy JA, Caldwell-Brown D, Lin AN, et al. Mupirocin-resistant *Staphylococcus aureus* after long-term treatment of patients with epidermolysis bullosa. J Am Acad Dermatol 1990;22:893–5.

[35] Cohen PR, Grossman ME. Management of cutaneous lesions associated with an emerging epidemic: community-acquired methicillin-resistant *Staphylococcus aureus* skin infections. J Am Acad Dermatol 2004;51:132–5.

[36] Eliopoulos GM. Mechanisms of bacterial resistance to antimicrobial drugs. In: Gorbach SL, Bartlett JG, Blacklow NR, editors. Infectious diseases. 2nd edition. Philadelphia: WB Saunders; 1998. p. 319–30.

[37] Del Rosso JQ. Cephalosporin antibiotics. Dis Mon 2004;50:315–31.

[38] Del Rosso JQ, Webster GF, Jackson M, et al. Two randomized phase III clinical trials evaluating anti-inflammatory dose doxycycline (40 mg doxycycline, USP capsules) administered once daily treatment for rosacea. J Am Acad Dermatol 2004, accepted for publication.

[39] Skidmore RS, Kovack R, Walker C, et al. Effects of subantimicrobial-dose doxycycline in the treatment of moderate acne. Arch Dermatol 2003;139: 459–64.

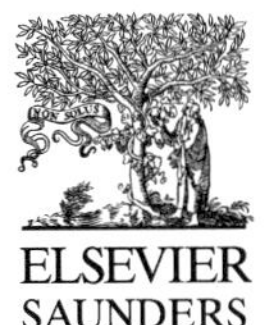

ELSEVIER
SAUNDERS

Dermatol Clin 25 (2007) 133–135

DERMATOLOGIC
CLINICS

Anti-Inflammatory Activity of Tetracyclines

Guy Webster, MD, PhD[a],*, James Q. Del Rosso, DO, FAOCD[b]

[a]Department of Dermatology, Jefferson Medical College, 833 Chestnut Street, Philadelphia, PA 19107, USA
[b]Valley Hospital Medical Center, PMB-531, 3230 E. Flamingo Rad #8, Las Vegas, NV 89121, USA

The tetracycline family of drugs has activity in diverse diseases and multiple mechanisms. Originally developed in the 1950s as antibacterial antibiotics, the tetracyclines are now known to exhibit multiple significant anti-inflammatory actions. The anti-inflammatory activity was probably first suspected by dermatologists who observed improvement in rosacea, a disorder not shown to be associated with a causative bacterium, and improvement in acne out of proportion to the decrease in populations of *Propionibacterium acnes*.

Mechanisms of anti-inflammatory activity

Indirect activity

Tetracycline, doxycycline, and minocycline are capable of rendering normal bacterial flora less inflammatory by inhibiting bacterial products that stimulate inflammation. Extremely low antibiotic concentrations—that is, concentrations that are beneath the minimal inhibitory concentration of *P acnes* and that have no effect on the bacterial growth curve—cause the organism to produce lower amounts of neutrophil chemoattractants, such as peptide chemotactic factor and lipase [1,2]. Thus, even without reducing bacterial numbers, tetracyclines may modulate improvement in inflammatory disease induced by bacteria.

Direct anti-inflammatory activity

Inhibition of chemotaxis

White blood cell migration is an early event in the inflammatory process. Tetracyclines have been shown to inhibit white cell movement both in vitro and in skin window experiments in vivo [3–5]. The mechanism of inhibition involves chelation of intracellular calcium, the availability of which is critical for the assembly of the microtubules that influence cell movement [6].

Inhibition of granuloma formation

Tetracyclines have substantial inhibitory activity in a model of granuloma formation in which human peripheral blood mononuclear cells are incubated with dextrin beads that serve as the nidus for formation of granulomalike structures [7]. Among tetracycline derivatives, tetracycline-mediated inhibition was 10 fold weaker than that of doxycycline and minocycline, which were active at pharmacologically achievable dosages. Other commonly used antibiotics, such as ampicillin and erythromycin, were inactive in the system. The mechanism of the inhibition is uncertain but may relate to inhibition of protein kinase C, an enzyme involved in signal transduction and control of inflammation. The activity in protein kinase C inhibition was proportional to the activity in the granuloma assay for each antibiotic.

Protease inhibition

Tetracyclines inhibit matrix metalloproteases (MMPs), which are zinc-dependant enzymes that are involved in many inflammatory diseases, wound healing, embryogenesis, tumor invasion, and angiogenesis.

Recent work suggests that ocular rosacea and other corneal surface diseases are mediated by MMPs in tear fluid. Maata and colleagues [8] found that tear fluid MMP-8 is elevated in rosacea in proportion to disease activity and that doxycycline therapy alleviates symptoms of rosacea and lowers MMP-8 levels. Kim and colleagues [9] have further shown that doxycycline interferes

___

* Corresponding author. Suite 10, 720 Yorklyn Road, Hockessin, DE 19707.

E-mail address: gfweb@earthlink.net (G. Webster).

doi:10.1016/j.det.2007.01.012

derm.theclinics.com

with TGF-beta-1–induced MMP-9 production in corneal epithelial cells, suggesting a mechanism for its activity in ocular rosacea.

Protease inhibition is also involved in the beneficial effects of doxycycline on chronic periodontal disease. Doses of subantimicrobial doxycline, while having no effect on the gingival microflora, even after prolonged administration over several months, demonstrate positive therapeutic effects on the course of chronic periodontitis. This activity has been linked to MMP inhibition [10,11].

Angiogenesis and metastasis are also linked to MMP activity. In several models, doxycycline and the nonantibiotic analog, incyclinide, have been found active in suppressing MMP-linked central nervous system angiogenesis and bony tumor growth [12,13]. Vascular tumors also respond to this approach. Most notably, 41% of patients with advanced Kaposi's sarcoma experienced significant regression of disease when treated with incyclinide [14].

Apoptosis has been both increased and decreased by tetracyclines in various experimental model systems through effects on capsases, enzymcs that may activate apoptosis [15 17]. The exact role that this activity might play in vivo is uncertain.

Activity in inflammatory diseases

Doxycycline and minocycline use has been sporadically reported in many inflammatory diseases in the form of case reports and short series. The drugs have proven to be particularly useful in a few diseases.

Acne vulgaris

Subantimicrobial doses of doxycycline administered over a 6-month period have been shown to reduce inflammatory and noninflammatory acne lesions in patients with acne vulgaris of moderate severity [18].

Rosacea

Anti-inflammatory dose doxycycline, administered as a 40-mg controlled-release capsule once daily, has been shown to reduce inflammatory lesions and erythema in patients with papulopustular rosacea [19]. This specific formulation, approved by the Food and Drug Administration for treatment of rosacea, demonstrates pharmacokinetic properties that allow for anti-inflammatory

activity without antibiotic effects, provided administration is once daily.

Bullous dermatoses

Autoimmune inflammatory diseases, such as bullous pemphigoid and pemphigus, have shown clear beneficial responses to treatment with tetracyclines [20]. A number of semianecdotal reports have accumulated that document the effects of the drug, but there is no definitive well-controlled study to document efficacy. The mechanism is uncertain and may be a combination of antineutrophil effects and inhibition of proteases. Typically, doxycycline is used as a steroid-sparing agent and has proven to be most useful in bullous pemphigoid that has been brought initially under control with prednisone. The authors have had a number of patients who have been completely controlled on doxycycline for several years, with subsequent recurrence of disease when the drug was discontinued.

Granulomatous diseases

The in vitro granuloma-inhibitory activity of tetracyclines suggests that they may be of use in granulomatous disease. Two reports show benefit, one on ulcerative sarcoidosis lesions [21] of the leg and the other on sarcoidal parotitis [22]. Other granulomatous diseases, including silica granulomas [23] and granulomatous cheilitis [24], have been reported to respond to tetracyclines. Webster, the lead author of this article, has treated numerous patients with sarcoidosis using minocycline and found that those with leg lesions show the clearest benefit.

Box 1. Nonantibiotic activities of tetracyclines

Indirect
   Reduction of *P acnes*
   Inhibition of lipase production
   Inhibition of chemotactic factor
     production

Direct
   Inhibition of leukocyte movement
   Inhibition of protein kinase C
   Inhibition of granuloma formation
   Inhibition of proteases
     Anti-angiogenic activity
     Anti-metastatic activity

Livedo vasculitis

The lead author has treated a number of chronically ulcerated livedo vasculitis patients with doxycycline and has had notable success in several instances. About 50% of patients have ulcers that completely heal on 100 mg twice daily, and have recurrence of ulceration when the medication is discontinued.

Summary

It appears that anti-inflammatory uses of tetracyclines are just beginning to be understood. Incyclinide, a chemically modified doxycycline with no antibiotic activity but enhanced anti-inflammatory activity is a tantalizing example of what might be possible for treatment of dermatologic disorders, such as acne vulgaris. More extensive and organized study of the effects of tetracyclines on metastasis and neurological disease would seem to be relatively uncomplicated to perform given the benign side-effect profile of the drugs and their availability (Box 1).

References

[1] Webster GF, McGinley KJ, Leyden JJ. Inhibition of lipase production in *Propionibacterium acnes* by sub-minimal inhibitory concentrations of tetracyclines and erythromycin. Br J Dermatol 1981;104:453–7.

[2] Webster GF, Leyden JJ, McGinley KJ, et al. Suppression of polymorphonuclear leukocyte chemotactic factor production in *Propionibacterium acnes* by sub-minimal inhibitory concentrations of tetracyclines and erythromycin. Antimicrob Agents Chemother 1982;21:770–2.

[3] Esterly NB, Furey NL, Flannagan LE. The effect of antimicrobial agents on chemotaxis. J Invest Dermatol 1978;70:51–5.

[4] Esterly NB, Kovansky JS, Furey NS, et al. Neutrophil chemotaxis in patients with acne receiving tetracycline. Arch Dermatol 1984;120:1308–13.

[5] Gabler WL, Creamer HR. Suppression of human neutrophil functions by tetracycline. J Periodontal Res 1991;26:52–8.

[6] Goodheart GL. Further evidence of the role of bivalent cations in leukocyte chemotaxis. J Reticuloendothel Soc 1979;25:545–54.

[7] Webster GF, Toso SM, Hegemann LR. Inhibition of *in vitro* granuloma formation by tetracyclines and ciprofloxacin: involvement of protein kinase C. Arch Dermatol 1994;130:748–52.

[8] Maata M, Kari O, Tervahartiala T, et al. Tera fluid levels of MMP-8 are elevated in ocular rosacea—treatment effect of oral doxycycline. Graefes Arch Clin Exp Ophthalmol 2006;244:957–62.

[9] Kim HS, Luo L, Pflugfelder SC, et al. Doxycycline inhibits TGF-beta-1 induced MMP-9 via Smad and MAPK pathways in cultured human corneal epithelial cells. Invest Ophthalmol Vis Sci 2005;46:840–8.

[10] Golub LM, Ramamurthy NS, Mcnamara TF, et al. Tetracyclines inhibit tissue collagenase activity a new mechanism in the treatment of periodontal disease. J Periodontal Res 1984;19:651–5.

[11] Ciancio S, Ashley R. Safety and efficacy of sub-antimicrobial doxycycline therapy in patients with adult periodontitis. Adv Dent Res 1998;12:27–37.

[12] Lee CZ, Xu HB, Hashimoto T, et al. Doxycycline suppresses cerebral MMP-9 and angiogenesis induced by focal hyperstimulation of vascular endothelial growth factor in a mouse model. Stroke 2004;35:1715–9.

[13] Saikali Z, Singh G. Doxycycline and other tetracyclines in the treatment of bone metastasis. Anticancer Drugs 2004;14:773–8.

[14] Dezube BJ, Krown SE, Lee JY, et al. Randomized phase II trial of matrix metalloproteinase inhibitor col-3 in AIDS-related Kaposi's sarcoma. J Clin Oncol 2006;24:1389–94.

[15] Onoda T, Ono T, Dhar DK, et al. Tetracycline analogs (doxycycline and col-3) induce caspase dependant and independent apoptosis in human cancer cells. Int J Cancer 2006;118:1309–15.

[16] Sanchez-Mejia RO, Ona VO, Friedlander RM. Minocycline reduces traumatic brain injury–mediated caspase 1 activation tissue damage, and neurological dysfunction. Neurosurgery 2001;28:1393–401.

[17] Chen M, Ona VO, Mingwei L, et al. Minocycline inhibits caspase 1 and caspase 3 expression and delays mortality in a transgenic mouse model of Huntington disease. Nat Med 2000;6:797–801.

[18] Skidmore R, Kovach R, Walker C, et al. Effects of subantimicrobial-dose doxycycline in the treatment of moderate acne. Arch Dermatol 2003;139:459–64.

[19] Del Rosso JQ, Webster GF, Jackson M, et al. Two randomized phase III clinical trials evaluating anti-inflammatory dose doxycycline (40-mg doxycycline USP capsules) administered once daily for treatment of rosacea. J Am Acad Dermatol, in press.

[20] Sapadin AN, Fleischmajer R. Tetracyclines: nonantibiotic properties and their clinical implications. J Am Acad Dermatol 2006;54:258–65.

[21] Bachelez H, Senet P, Cadranel J, et al. The use of tetracyclines for treatment of sarcoidosis. Arch Dermatol 2001;137:69–73.

[22] Ohtsuka S, Yanadori A, Tabata H, et al. Sarcoidosis with giant parotomegaly. Cutis 2001;68:199–200.

[23] Senet P, Bachelez H, Olivaud L, et al. Minocycline for the treatment of cutaneous silica granulomas. Br J Dermatol 1999;140:985–7.

[24] Veller-Formosa C, Catalano P, Peserico A. Minocycline in granulomatous cheilitis: experience with six cases. Dermatology 1992;185:220–2.

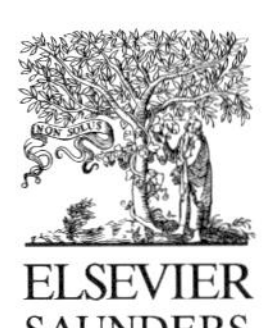

ELSEVIER
SAUNDERS

Dermatol Clin 25 (2007) 137–146

DERMATOLOGIC
CLINICS

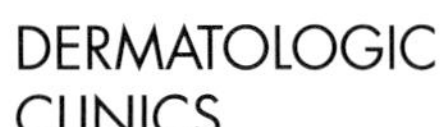

Pharmacologic Modulation of Sebaceous Gland Activity: Mechanisms and Clinical Applications

Shari B. Clarke, MD[a], Amanda M. Nelson, PhD[b],
Rosalyn E. George, MD[a], Diane M. Thiboutot, MD[a,b,]*

[a]*The Department of Dermatology, The Pennsylvania State University College of Medicine,
P.O. Box 850, Hershey, PA 17033, USA*
[b]*The Jake Gittlen Cancer Research Foundation, The Pennsylvania State University College of Medicine,
C7801 BMR Building, MC H059, 500 University Drive, Hershey, PA 17033, USA*

Acne vulgaris is one of the most prevalent skin conditions encountered by dermatologists, affecting nearly 85% of people between the ages of 12 and 24 years, and 40 to 50 million people in the United States each year [1–3]. Acne is a multifactorial disease that affects the pilosebaceous unit and the complicated interaction of four main pathogenic factors leads to its development. These include (1) the production of sebum by androgen-mediated stimulation of sebaceous glands, (2) abnormal hyperkeratinization of the follicles leading to follicular plugging and comedone formation, (3) colonization of the pilosebaceous unit by the gram-positive bacteria *Propionibacterium acnes*, and (4) stimulation of an inflammatory cascade and release of inflammatory mediators by *P acnes* into the follicle and surrounding dermis [4].

The pilosebaceous unit is composed of four distinct components, including the hair follicle itself, the keratinized follicular infundibulum that sheds corneocytes into the lumen, the sebaceous gland, and the sebaceous duct that connects the gland to the infundibulum. Sebaceous glands and holocrine sebum production are regulated primarily by hormonal stimulation, especially the androgen dihydrotestosterone (DHT). Sebaceous glands are present at birth with sebum production being

relatively high during the first 6 months of life. After 6 months however, sebum production declines and remains low until puberty, when sebaceous gland activity increases dramatically and remains stable through adulthood. The number, size, and activity of sebaceous glands are thought to be inherited with the number remaining fairly stable throughout life whereas the size increases with age.

Acne begins with the formation of the microcomedone and the severity of acne is based on the type, number, and distribution of lesions, as well as whether or not scarring is present. Mild acne is composed mostly of open and closed comedones that are produced when corneocytes are retained and accumulate in the infundibulum, leading to hyperkeratosis. Moderate acne is characterized by comedone formation but also moderate numbers of papules and pustules, formed following the rupture of comedones and subsequent *P acnes* proliferation and inflammation. Moderately severe acne is composed of more numerous papules, pustules, and comedones as well as a few nodular lesions affecting the face, chest, and back. Finally, severe or nodulocystic acne has many painful nodular lesions as well as smaller papules, pustules, and comedones, and histologically marked scarring and inflammation are evident.

There are multiple available medications for the treatment of acne, and therapy is usually based on the severity of lesions. Topical retinoids are the mainstays of acne treatment, and can be combined with antimicrobials (eg, benzoyl

* Corresponding author. Department of Dermatology, Penn State University College of Medicine, P.O. Box 850, Hershey, PA 17033.
E-mail address: dthiboutot@psu.edu
(D.M. Thiboutot).

peroxide) and an oral or topical antibiotic. If the acne is mild, topical therapy alone may be sufficient, with the addition of systemic agents being required for moderate to severe acne that does not respond to topicals. Given the extensive research that supports the role of the sebaceous gland in the development of acne, specific therapies have been developed that target the sebaceous gland, in particular by decreasing sebum production, both directly and indirectly. Only isotretinoin and hormonal therapy, such as oral contraceptives and anti-androgens, play a significant role in inhibiting sebaceous gland activity (Table 1).

Isotretinoin

Isotretinoin or 13-*cis* retinoic acid, is a synthetic vitamin A (retinol) analog first approved by the US Food and Drug Administration (FDA) in 1982 for the treatment of severe recalcitrant nodulocystic acne [5]. Although initially developed for that purpose, isotretinoin has been used more recently for patients with moderate and moderately severe acne who are unresponsive to conventional therapies [6]. The half-life is 22 hours and the bioavailability, which can be increased by taking isotretinoin with food, is 25%. Isotretinoin therapy has been shown to improve psychological distress (anxiety and depressive symptoms) as well as reduce scarring in acne patients [7]. Isotretinoin acts primarily by decreasing the size of the sebaceous glands and reducing sebum production by up to 90%, thereby inhibiting the growth of *P acnes* and subsequent inflammation. In addition, like topical retinoids, it inhibits comedone formation by normalizing follicular keratinization.

Mechanism of action

Isotretinoin is the only oral retinoid known to have profound effect on sebaceous gland activity, although the exact mechanisms remain elusive. Evidence supports the fact that isotretinoin can influence each of the four factors involved in the pathogenesis of acne by influencing cell-cycle progression, cellular differentiation, cell survival, and apoptosis.

Unlike tretinoin (all-*trans* retinoic acid [ATRA]), isotretinoin has little to no ability to bind to cellular retinol-binding proteins or the retinoic acid nuclear receptors (RARs and RXRs) [8–10]. Instead, it may act as a pro-drug that is converted intracellularly to ATRA and 9-*cis* RA, which are agonists for RAR nuclear receptors and both RAR and RXR nuclear receptors, respectively [9,11]. It is well established, however, that isotretinoin is superior to either 9-*cis* RA or ATRA for suppression of sebaceous gland activity and sebum production [11–13]. Another proposed theory is that isotretinoin may act in a receptor independent manner, influencing cellular signaling pathways by either direct protein interactions, as demonstrated with other retinoids, or by enzyme inhibition [14–17].

The primary change within the sebaceous follicle in acne is an alteration in follicular keratinization; isotretinoin may decrease hyperkeratinization by

Table 1
Acne medications effecting sebum production

Drug	Dose	Side effects
Oral retinoids		
Isotretinoin	0.5–1.0 mg/kg/day cumulative 120 mg/kg	Teratatogenicity, mood changes, elevated liver enzymes, hypertriglyceridemia, cheilitis, xerosis, visual disturbances, pseudotumor cerebri, arthralgias
Hormonal agents		
Spironolactone	50–200 mg daily[b]	Menstrual irregularities[c], diuretic effect hyperkalemia, breast tenderness, decreased libido, feminization of male fetus
Cyproterone acetate	2–100 mg daily[a]	Similar to spironolactone
Flutamide	250 mg twice daily	Severe hepatitis, teratogenicity
Oral contraceptives	Daily	Thromboembolism, migraine cephalgia, menstrual irregularities

[a] May be effective at lower doses, not available in the United States.
[b] Usually combined with oral contraceptives.
[c] Less common when combined with oral contraceptives.

50% [18,19]. The exact mechanism is unknown, but research demonstrates that isotretinoin does not affect the metabolic activity of the keratinocytes [20].

Of all of the treatments available for acne, isotretinoin is the most potent inhibitor of sebum production. Histologically, a drastic decrease in the size, shape, and lipid content of sebaceous glands is seen after 16 weeks of isotretinoin therapy [21]. These effects may be explained by cell-cycle arrest or apoptosis [22]. Further studies indicate that isotretinoin influences the G1/S phase of the cell cycle as evidenced by decreased DNA synthesis, increased p21 protein, and decreased cyclin D1 protein. In addition, isotretinoin induces apoptosis in sebocytes and these effects are independent of RAR receptor activation [22]. It seems likely that the decrease in sebum production may be the net result of sebaceous gland involution in response to isotretinoin treatment. Future experiments are needed to confirm this hypothesis. Furthermore, isotretinoin has been shown to competitively inhibit the 3α-hydroxysteroid activity of retinol dehydrogenase leading to decreased androgen synthesis in vitro [17,23].

The predominant organism in the follicular flora is *P acnes*. Isotretinoin significantly reduces the number of *P acnes*, including antibiotic-resistant strains, with levels slowly returning to baseline after discontinuing therapy [24,25]. The exact mechanism of isotretinoin's effect on *P acnes* is unknown, but may be accomplished directly by targeting *P acnes*, indirectly by decreasing sebum production thereby removing their food supply, or, as in the case with ATRA, by increasing host defense mechanisms [26].

P acnes plays an important role in the production of inflammatory acne by stimulating the classical and alternative complement pathways [27]. *P acnes* releases a variety of lytic enzymes and cytokines that are chemotactic for inflammatory cells. With the reduction of *P acnes* with isotretinoin treatment, inflammation is likely to diminish. In addition, isotretinoin inhibits the migration of polymorphonuclear leukocytes into the skin supporting its role in the reduction of inflammation that is associated with acne [23].

Clinical applications

In addition to its proven benefit in the treatment of nodulocystic acne, isotretinoin has been used successfully to treat, although sometimes only temporarily, other acneiform conditions, such as solid facial edema (Morbihan's disease), and gram-negative folliculitis, as well as disorders of cornification and as chemoprophylaxis of skin cancer in patients with defective DNA repair [28–33]. This includes patients with basal cell nevus syndrome (Gorlin syndrome), xeroderma pigmentosum, and inhibiting eruptive keratoacanthomas [34–36]. Interestingly, isotretinoin's benefits span most fields of medicine, including its successful use in treating renal cell cancer, prostate cancer, recurrent malignant gliomas, and spinal cord astrocytomas among other visceral malignancies [31,37–42].

Dosing

Traditionally, when being used for acne, isotretinoin has been prescribed at a dose of 0.5 to 1.0 mg/kg per day for 4 to 6 months, to reach a cumulative dose of 120 mg/kg [43]. Recently, low-dose isotretinoin at 20 mg per day for 6 months has been used to treat patients with moderate acne with nearly 95% achieving significant improvement or complete remission. The relapse rate was between 4% and 6%, with a mean total dose of 66 to 70 mg/kg at the end of 6 months [6]. The most common side effects in this study were mild cheilitis and xerosis.

Of all patients treated with isotretinoin, approximately 40% of patients are acne free at the end of the treatment period, whereas another 40% have a recurrence that responds to medications previously tried. The remaining 20% will require a second course of isotretinoin. Patients more likely to relapse include those younger than 16 years of age, adult females, and those with significant truncal involvement [44]. For the most severe cases, patients may initially be started at a dose of 0.5 mg/kg daily for the first month to prevent a significant acne flare and then increased over the next month to 1.0 mg/kg daily. In addition, simultaneous administration of prednisone may be helpful in cases of acne fulminans or in those with a severe initial flare.

Side effects

Multiple mucocutaneous and systemic side effects have been described with isotretinoin use and the observed side effects are usually dose dependent and reversible. Many side effects are similar to those seen in hypervitaminosis A, since isotretinoin is a vitamin A analog. Cheilitis is by far the most common symptom, occurring in nearly 100% of patients treated, and noncompliance should be suspected in the absence of cheilitis [31]. Xerosis is another frequent side effect and the continual use of topical emollients is recommended to treat both the cheilitis and xerosis.

Other reported side effects include hyperostoses, xerophthalmia, blurry vision, nyctalopia (night blindness), headache, fatigue, myalgias, hyperlipidemia, skin atrophy, fragility, excessive formation of granulation tissue for up to 6 months following completion of therapy, hair and nail brittleness (more common with acetretin), and acne fulminans, which requires prompt discontinuation of treatment and initiation of systemic corticosteroids. A potentially serious side effect that all patients should be warned about is the development of pseudotumor cerebri, or benign intracranial hypertension. It has been reported more commonly with the coadministration of tetracyclines, which are also known to cause pseudotumor cerebri. Symptoms include severe persistent headache, blurred vision, nausea, and vomiting [31]. Patients experiencing any of these symptoms should be advised to promptly discontinue isotretinoin therapy and seek medical attention.

Although some reports suggest that alpha tocopherol (Vitamin E) may ameliorate toxicities related to retinoid use (particularly in patients with myelodysplastic syndrome), other studies have found no difference in the incidence and severity of side effects in patients treated with alpha tocopherol [45]. Further studies may be needed to more clearly delineate the utility of alpha tocopherol in the relief of retinoid-induced symptoms.

In 1998, a label warning about depression and suicide was added to isotretinoin and the issue of depression and suicidal behavior in acne patients treated with isotretinoin is still an issue of great concern to many patients and parents. Between 1982 and 2000, the FDA received reports through its Adverse Event Reporting System of 431 cases of depression, suicidal ideation, suicide attempts, or suicide in patients treated with isotretinoin. There were 37 patients who committed suicide, 24 of them while using isotretinoin and 110 patients were hospitalized for depression, suicidal ideation, or suicide attempts. However, this risk does not seem to be higher than what would be predicted for the general population based on suicide rates in the United States [46]. A more recent meta-analysis showed similar rates of depression among isotretinoin users and those taking oral antibiotics (control group), ranging from 1% to 11%. Some studies have even discovered a trend toward less severe depressive symptoms following isotretinoin therapy [47]. Further studies are needed to elucidate a true causal relationship between isotretinoin and depressive symptoms or suicide. A careful assessment for depression and suicidal ideation should to be conducted on all patients currently using isotretinoin as well as those being considered for therapy.

The most concerning systemic side effect of isotretinoin is its potential teratogenicity. Isotretinoin remains in the circulation for 1 month following discontinuation of therapy. A single dose of isotretinoin during the first trimester carries a 20% to 25 % risk of major fetal malformation [48,49]. In 36 prospectively observed pregnancies, 8 were associated with spontaneous abortion and 5 had serious congenital malformations [49]. This constellation of birth defects is known as retinoic acid embryopathy, which is characterized by external ear abnormalities (anotia/microtia), craniofacial abnormalities (micrognathia, cleft palate), cardiovascular abnormalities (conotruncal heart defects and aortic arch abnormalities), thymus gland abnormalities, ophthalmic abnormalities (microphthalmia, retinal or optic nerve defects), and central nervous system malformations (hydrocephalus and microcephaly) [49]. Severe disturbances in the migration of neural crest cells during embryogenesis are believed to play a key role in the mechanism of retinoic acid teratogenicity [50].

Despite the implementation of various pregnancy prevention programs, a pregnancy rate among women undergoing isotretinoin therapy of 3.4 per 1000 courses of isotretinoin has been reported [31]. Because of this unacceptably high rate of pregnancies, a national isotretinoin registry named iPLEDGE (www.iPLEDGEprogram.com) was mandated by the FDA and put into effect on March 1, 2006, to more tightly protect against inadvertent pregnancies and document those cases that do occur.

Hormonal therapy

Androgens, in particular dihydrotestosterone (DHT), play an important role in the pathophysiology of acne. Although the exact mechanisms are still under investigation, androgens act primarily by stimulating sebum production by the sebaceous glands. This is supported by evidence that patients lacking functional androgen receptors do not produce sebum or develop acne, and that systemic administration of testosterone and dihydroepiandosterone increases the size and function of sebaceous glands [51].

The major androgens that interact with the androgen receptor are testosterone and DHT, with DHT being 5 to 10 times more potent than testosterone. Androgen receptors have been localized to both the keratinocytes of the outer root sheath of hair follicles as well as the basal layer of the sebaceous gland. Most androgens are produced in peripheral tissues, principally the adrenal glands and the gonads, with only a small percentage being produced by the sebaceous glands themselves. The weaker androgens, DHEAS (adrenal origin) and androstenedione (ovarian origin) are converted in the skin to testosterone and DHT. The type 1 isozyme of the enzyme 5α-reductase, located within the sebaceous gland, catalyzes the conversion of testosterone to the more potent DHT within the skin [52]. In men, DHT is derived mostly from testosterone, whereas in women DHT is derived from androstenedione.

Endocrine evaluation

It is evident that hormones influence the development of acne; however, the majority of patients with acne do not have an endocrine abnormality. Such an abnormality should be suspected in patients with sudden onset of severe acne, hirsutism, irregular menstrual periods, and signs or symptoms of hyperandrogenism such as increased libido, acanthosis nigricans, cushingoid features, deepening of the voice, or androgenic alopecia [53]. In addition to acne, these patients may develop insulin resistance and are at risk for the development of diabetes mellitus and cardiovascular disease.

When a female patient is suspected of having an underlying endocrine abnormality, screening tests for androgen excess may be helpful in determining the source of androgens. These include DHEAS, total testosterone, free testosterone, and luteinizing hormone/follicle stimulating hormone (LH/FSH) ratio. An elevated DHEAS is indicative of either an adrenal tumor (>8000 ng/mL) or congenital adrenal hyperplasia (4000 to 8000 ng/mL) (Fig. 1). An elevated total testosterone points toward either an ovarian tumor (>150 to 200 ng/dL) or polycystic ovary disease (mild elevations). Finally, an elevated LH/FSH ratio supports a diagnosis of polycystic ovary disease. In cases of suspected congenital adrenal hyperplasia, an elevated 17-hydroxyprogesterone level confirms an adrenal source of androgens. It is important that these tests be conducted at a time apart from ovulation such as just before or during the menstrual period and that oral contraceptives should be discontinued 4 to 6 weeks before the evaluation [2]. All abnormal results should be confirmed with repeat testing. Even when all laboratory evaluation is negative, there may still be a role for hormonal therapy particularly in women whose acne tends to flare around the

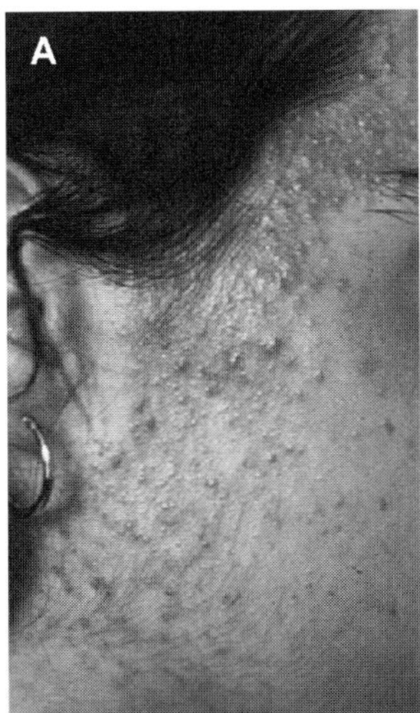
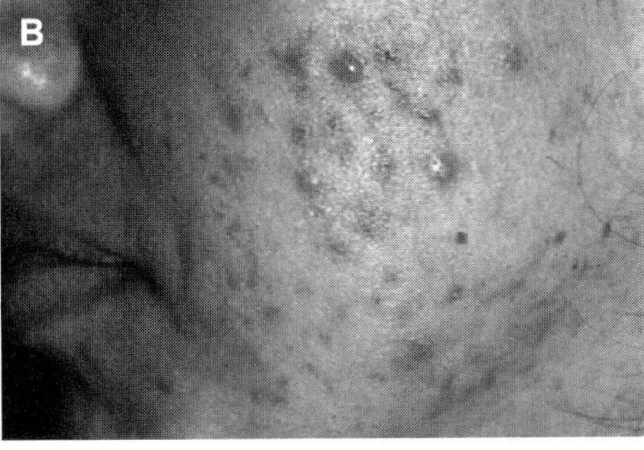

Fig. 1. Hormonal acne. (*A*) Acne secondary to an adrenal tumor. This 10-year-old female patient developed acne and hirsutism as a result of an androgen-producing adrenal tumor. (*B*) Acne associated with congenital adrenal hyperplasia.

time of menses, as these patients have higher serum levels of DHEAS, DHT, and testosterone when compared with women without acne [54].

Agents for hormonal therapy

When deciding to commence hormonal therapy for a female patient, two main classes of drugs should be considered. The first group is the androgen receptor blocks, or anti-androgens, which block the effect of androgens on the sebaceous gland and the follicular infundibulum. The classic example is spironolactone. The second group is the inhibitors of androgen production, both by the adrenal gland and ovary. Oral contraceptives are the archetype for this group.

Androgen receptor blockers

Spironolactone. Spironolactone is a steroidal androgen receptor blocker that has been used for over 20 years for the treatment of acne and hirsutism [55,56]. The mechanism by which spironolactone is believed to work is by decreasing sebum production and inhibiting type 2 17β-hydroxysteroid dehydrogenase, thereby inhibiting the conversion of androstenedione to testosterone [57,58]. Additional mechanisms include the inhibition of 5α-reductase and elevation of steroid hormone–binding globulin [59]. This results in a 30% to 50% decrease in sebum excretion rate. Spironolactone is also an aldosterone antagonist and diuretic [60]. In men, spironolactone is poorly tolerated because of gynecomastia and decreased libido and therefore should only be used in women for the treatment of acne [56].

The usual dosage for the treatment of acne is 50 to 200 mg daily. However, lower daily doses may be effective in controlling acne with the advantage of having a reduced side effect profile. In 85 women treated with 50 to 100 mg daily of spironolactone, 33% experienced complete clearance with an additional 33% having marked improvement; only 40% of patients reported side effects [61]. In contrast, another study demonstrated that 91% of patients who received 200 mg of spironolactone daily reported side effects [61,62]. Doses as low as 25 mg twice daily or even once daily often produce good clinical response and are well tolerated in most women [53]. Following success with orally administered spironolactone, topical spironolactone was investigated for its ability to also reduce sebum secretion. When topical 5% spironolactone gel was compared with vehicle gel in a split face trial, a significant reduction in the rate of sebum secretion

was seen at 12 weeks (4 weeks after termination of application), but not at 8 weeks (end of treatment) on the treated side when compared with the untreated side [63]. Other evidence has not supported this finding.

Spironolactone has multiple associated side effects; however, long-term safety for its use in acne has been reported, although this drug is not approved by the FDA for this indication [55]. Most women treated with spironolactone experience at least one side effect and these are thought to be dose dependent [61]. The most common side effect is menstrual irregularities, primarily metrorrhagia, amenorrhea, break-through bleeding, and shortened length of menstrual cycle, which can be ameliorated by lowering the dose or concomitant use of oral contraceptives [56,64]. Other common side effects are breast tenderness or enlargement, headache, fatigue, dizziness, lightheadedness, diuretic effect, orthostatic hypotension, hyperkalemia, and decreased libido [56,61]. Serum electrolytes should be monitored in older women with additional medical problems, when higher doses are required, and with coadministration of oral contraceptives containing the progestin drosperinone [53]. It is important to avoid pregnancy during therapy with spironolactone as well as other anti-androgens because of the risk of abnormalities of the male genitalia including hypospadias and feminization of the male fetus [65].

Cyproterone acetate. Cyproterone acetate is a progestin that acts as an androgen receptor blocker and inhibits ovulation. It is used in Canada, Europe, and Asia for the treatment of severe acne resistant to traditional therapy. Its effectiveness in the treatment of acne is related to its ability to reduce sebum production and perhaps comedogenesis [66]. It can be used as a sole agent or in a combination with an oral contraceptive. Diane-35 or Dianette (Schering) is the combination of 2 mg cyproterone acetate and ethinyl estradiol (35 to 50 μg). It is the only hormonal therapy whose sole indication is the treatment of acne [67]. When used alone, higher doses of 50 to 100 mg are given on days 5 to 14 of the menstrual cycle [68]. In various studies, a 75% to 90% reduction in acne lesion counts and severity has been observed [2,69].

Flutamide. Flutamide is a nonsteroidal androgen receptor blocker used in the treatment of prostate cancer [60]. It is converted to a potent metabolite 2-hydroxyflutamide, which inhibits the binding of dihydrotestosterone to androgen receptors. It can also be used in the treatment of acne, hirsutism, and androgenic alopecia [70]. It is effective at doses of 250 mg twice daily in combination with an oral contraceptive. Liver enzymes should be monitored during therapy, as fatal hepatitis has been reported [71]. Hepatotoxicity may be dose and age dependent, as low doses of 62.5 to 125 mg have been found to be safe and effective [72,73].

Androgen production blockers

This category can be divided into therapies that block production of androgens by the adrenal gland and those that block androgen production by the ovaries. These agents include glucocorticoids and oral contraceptives, respectively. Glucocorticoids, which inhibit adrenal androgen production, are most often used in the treatment of patients with congenital adrenal hyperplasia, where inherent defects in cortisol synthesis result in an accumulation of androgen precursors. Options include prednisone at low doses of 2.5 to 5 mg at bedtime or low-dose dexamethasone. Prednisone is the preferred agent because of increased risk of adrenal suppression with dexamethasone [53].

Androgen production from the ovaries can be inhibited by gonadotropin-releasing hormone agonists such as buserelin, nafarelin, or leuprolide. These agents inhibit both androgen and estrogen production by the ovaries by interrupting the cyclic release of FSH and LH from the pituitary gland. These drugs are effective in the treatment of hirsutism and acne in addition to their use in prostate cancer. They are available as injectables or nasal sprays. Patients may experience menopausal symptoms, osteopenia, and headaches as a result of hypoestrogenism.

Oral contraceptives can also decrease sebum production and can be an effective treatment for acne (Fig. 2). Oral contraceptives are formulated with two agents, an estrogen (most commonly ethinyl estradiol) and a progestin. Historically, oral contraceptives had a high concentration of estrogen in the range of 100 to 150 µg. At these high doses, estrogens act to suppress sebum production as well as increase sex hormone–binding globulin by the liver, which lowers circulating levels of free testosterone. Oral contraceptives also suppress ovulation, which results in a decrease in the ovarian production of androgens and subsequent decrease in sebum production. Within the sebaceous gland, estrogen receptors (ERα and ERβ) are expressed in both basal and differentiating sebocytes [74,75]. The major active estrogen is

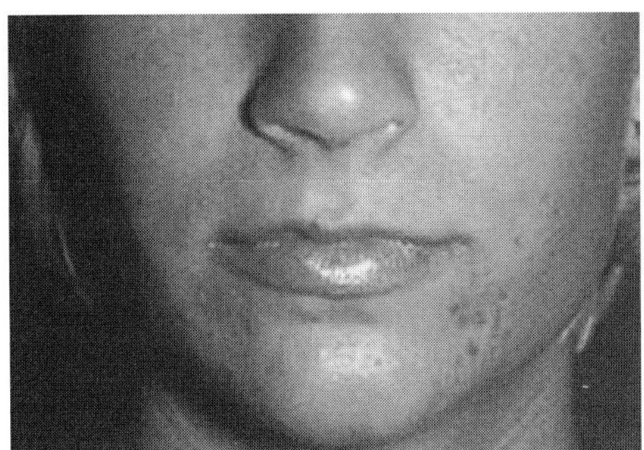

Fig. 2. Typical adult female acne.

estradiol, which is produced from testosterone by the action of the enzyme aromatase. Aromatase is active in the ovary, adipose tissue, and other peripheral tissues. Estradiol can be converted to the less potent estrogen, estrone by the action of the 17β-HSD enzyme. Both aromatase and 17β-HSD are present in the skin [76,77]. Estrogens regulate cell activities by binding to and activating estrogen receptors. Activation of cell surface receptors triggers signaling pathways, while nuclear hormone receptors bind to estrogen response elements leading to activation or suppression of gene transcription. Older formulations of oral contraceptives with the higher levels of estrogen have been replaced with newer generation oral contraceptives with estrogen ranging from 20 to 30 µg to reduce side effects.

The second component in oral contraceptives is the progestin. Like estrogens, progestins act through nuclear hormone receptors triggering activation or suppression of progesterone target genes leading to a cell-specific response. In the sebaceous gland, progesterone receptor B is expressed in both basal and differentiating sebocytes [78]. First- and second-generation progestins can react with the androgen receptor aggravating acne, hirsutism, and androgenic alopecia [79]. Newer third-generation progestins, such as norgestimate, desogestrel, and gestodene, are more selective for the progesterone receptor than the androgen receptor. In addition, progesterone has been shown to modulate pro-inflammatory and anti-inflammatory cytokines [80]. Whether progesterone receptor activation can lead to decreased inflammation in sebaceous glands is currently unknown. All oral contraceptives, regardless of their progestin, will to some degree inhibit serum androgen levels as well as increase sex hormone–binding globulin resulting in improvement in acne. Currently in the United States, there

Table 2
Oral contraceptives used in acne therapy

Drug	Estrogen (μg)	Progesterone (mg)
Ortho Tri-Cyclen[a]	Ethinyl estradiol 35	Norgestimate 0.18/0.215/0.25
Estrostep[a]	Ethinyl estradiol 20/30/35	Norethindrone 1
Yasmin	Ethinyl estradiol 30	Drospirenone 3
Aless	Ethinyl estradiol 20	Levonorgestrel 0.1
Mircette	Ethinyl estradiol 20/10	Desogestrel 0.15/0
Triphasil	Ethinyl estradiol 30/40/30	Levonorgestrel 0.5/0.75/0.125
Desogen	Ethinyl estradiol 30	Desogestrel 0.15
Ortho Cyclen	Ethinyl estradiol 35	Norgestimate 0.25

Limited to those studied in acne and available in the United States.
[a] FDA-approved for use in acne.

are only two oral contraceptives approved for use in the treatment of acne: 35 μg ethinyl estradiol/norgestimate (Ortho Tri-Cyclen) or 20 to 35 μg ethinyl estradiol/norethindrone acetate (Estrostep) (Table 2).

Drospirenone, a novel progestin derived from 17-alpha-spironolactone, possesses both anti-androgenic and anti-mineralocorticoid activity. The combination of drospirenone and 30 μg of ethinyl estradiol (Yasmin) has been shown to reduce inflammatory acne lesion counts by 60%, which were comparable to results seen with cyproterone acetate and ethinyl estradiol (Diane-35) [81].

Summary

One of the major factors in the pathogenesis of acne is sebum production. Of the countless therapies available for acne, only isotretinoin and hormonal therapy act to directly regulate the activity of the sebaceous gland. As more knowledge is gained about the complex functioning of the sebaceous gland, novel therapies will hopefully be developed to more effectively treat acne and reduce side effects.

References

[1] Fleischer AB Jr, Simpson JK, McMichael A, et al. Are there racial and sex differences in the use of oral isotretinoin for acne management in the United States? J Am Acad Dermatol 2003;49(4):662–6.

[2] Thiboutot DM. Endocrinological evaluation and hormonal therapy for women with difficult acne. J Eur Acad Dermatol Venereol 2001;15(Suppl 3): 57–61.

[3] James WD. Clinical practice. Acne. N Engl J Med 2005;352(14):1463–72.

[4] Haider A, Shaw JC. Treatment of acne vulgaris. JAMA 2004;292(6):726–35.

[5] Chia CY, Lane W, Chibnall J, et al. Isotretinoin therapy and mood changes in adolescents with moderate to severe acne: a cohort study. Arch Dermatol 2005;141(5):557–60.

[6] Amichai B, Shemer A, Grunwald MH. Low-dose isotretinoin in the treatment of acne vulgaris. J Am Acad Dermatol 2006;54(4):644–6.

[7] Rubinow DR, Peck GL, Squillace KM, et al. Reduced anxiety and depression in cystic acne patients after successful treatment with oral isotretinoin. J Am Acad Dermatol 1987;17(1):25–32.

[8] Fogh K, Voorhees JJ, Astrom A. Expression, purification, and binding properties of human cellular retinoic acid-binding protein type I and type II. Arch Biochem Biophys 1993;300(2):751–5.

[9] Allenby G, Bocquel MT, Saunders M, et al. Retinoic acid receptors and retinoid X receptors: interactions with endogenous retinoic acids. Proc Natl Acad Sci U S A 1993;90(1):30–4.

[10] Levin A, Bosakowski T, Kazmer S, et al. 13-cis retinoic acid does not bind to retinoic acid receptors alpha, beta and gamma. Toxicologist 1992;12:181.

[11] Ott F, Bollag W, Geiger JM. Oral 9-cis-retinoic acid versus 13-cis-retinoic acid in acne therapy. Dermatology 1996;193(2):124–6.

[12] Hommel L, Geiger JM, Harms M, et al. Sebum excretion rate in subjects treated with oral all-trans-retinoic acid. Dermatology 1996;193(2):127–30.

[13] Geiger J-M, Hommel L, Harms M, et al. Oral 13-cis retinoic acid is superior to 9-cis retinoic acid in sebo-suppression in human beings. J Am Acad Dermatol 1996;34(3):513–5.

[14] Zorn NE, Sauro MD. Retinoic acid induces translocation of protein kinase C (PKC) and activation of nuclear PKC (nPKC) in rat splenocytes. Int J Immunopharmacol 1995;17(4):303–11.

[15] Imam A, Hoyos B, Swenson C, et al. Retinoids as ligands and coactivators of protein kinase C alpha. FASEB J 2001;15(1):28–30.

[16] Hoyos B, Imam A, Chua R, et al. The cysteine-rich regions of the regulatory domains of Raf and protein kinase C as retinoid receptors. J Exp Med 2000; 192(6):835–45.

[17] Karlsson T, Vahlquist A, Kedishvili N, et al. 13-cis-retinoic acid competitively inhibits 3 alpha-hydroxysteroid oxidation by retinol dehydrogenase RoDH-4: a mechanism for its anti-androgenic effects in sebaceous glands? Biochem Biophys Res Commun 2003;303(1):273–8.

[18] Knutson DD. Ultrastructural observations in acne vulgaris: the normal sebaceous follicle and acne lesions. J Invest Dermatol 1974;62(3):288–307.

[19] Plewig G, Dressel H, Pfleger M, et al. Low dose isotretinoin combined with tretinoin is effective to correct abnormalities of acne. J Dtsch Dermatol Ges 2004;2(1):31–45.

[20] Dalziel K, Barton S, Marks R. The effects of isotretinoin on follicular and sebaceous gland differentiation. Br J Dermatol 1987;117(3):317–23.

[21] Goldstein JA, Socha-Szott A, Thomsen RJ, et al. Comparative effect of isotretinoin and etretinate on acne and sebaceous gland secretion. J Am Acad Dermatol 1982;6(4 Pt 2 Suppl):760–5.

[22] Nelson AM, Gilliland KL, Cong Z, et al. 13-cis retinoic acid induces apoptosis and cell cycle arrest in human SEB-1 sebocytes. J Invest Dermatol 2006;126(10):2178–89.

[23] Wozel G, Chang A, Zultak M, et al. The effect of topical retinoids on the leukotriene-B4-induced migration of polymorphonuclear leukocytes into human skin. Arch Dermatol Res 1991;283(3):158–61.

[24] Leyden JJ, McGinley KJ, Foglia AN. Qualitative and quantitative changes in cutaneous bacteria associated with systemic isotretinoin therapy for acne conglobata. J Invest Dermatol 1986;86(4):390–3.

[25] Coates P, Vyakrnam S, Ravenscroft JC, et al. Efficacy of oral isotretinoin in the control of skin and nasal colonization by antibiotic-resistant propionibacteria in patients with acne. Br J Dermatol 2005;153(6):1126–36.

[26] Seguin-Devaux C, Hanriot D, Dailloux M, et al. Retinoic acid amplifies the host immune response to LPS through increased T lymphocytes number and LPS binding protein expression. Mol Cell Endocrinol 2005;245(1–2):67–76.

[27] Webster GF. Complement activation in acne vulgaris. Consumption of complement by comedones. Infect Immun 1979;26:183–6.

[28] Mazzatenta C, Giorgino G, Rubegni P, et al. Solid persistent facial oedema (Morbihan's disease) following rosacea, successfully treated with isotretinoin and ketotifen. Br J Dermatol 1997;137(6):1020–1.

[29] Cunliffe WJ. Management of adult acne and acne variants. J Cutan Med Surg 1998;2(Suppl 3):7–13.

[30] Pelwig G. Acneiform dermatoses. Dermatology 1998;196:102–7.

[31] Ellis CN, Krach KJ. Uses and complications of isotretinoin therapy. J Am Acad Dermatol 2001;45(5):S150–7.

[32] Craven NM, Griffiths CE. Retinoids in the management of non-melanoma skin cancer and melanoma. Cancer Surv 1996;26:267–88.

[33] DiGiovanna JJ. Retinoid chemoprevention in the high-risk patient. J Am Acad Dermatol 1998;39(2 Pt 3):S82–5.

[34] Goldberg LH, Hsu SH, Alcalay J. Effectiveness of isotretinoin in preventing the appearance of basal cell carcinomas in basal cell nevus syndrome. J Am Acad Dermatol 1989;21(1):144–5.

[35] Kraemer KH, DiGiovanna JJ, Moshell AN, et al. Prevention of skin cancer in xeroderma pigmentosum with the use of oral isotretinoin. N Engl J Med 1988;318(25):1633–7.

[36] Schaller M, Korting HC, Wolff H, et al. Multiple keratoacanthomas, giant keratoacanthoma and keratoacanthoma centrifugum marginatum: development in a single patient and treatment with oral isotretinoin. Acta Derm Venereol 1996;76(1): 40–2.

[37] Motzer RJ, Schwartz L, Law TM, et al. Interferon alfa-2a and 13-cis-retinoic acid in renal cell carcinoma: antitumor activity in a phase II trial and interactions in vitro. J Clin Oncol 1995;13(8):1950–7.

[38] Stadler WM, Kuzel T, Dumas M, et al. Multicenter phase II trial of interleukin-2, interferon-alpha, and 13-cis-retinoic acid in patients with metastatic renal-cell carcinoma. J Clin Oncol 1998;16(5):1820–5.

[39] DiPaola RS, Weiss RE, Cummings KB, et al. Effect of 13-cis-retinoic acid and alpha-interferon on transforming growth factor beta1 in patients with rising prostate-specific antigen. Clin Cancer Res 1997; 3(11):1999–2004.

[40] Yung WK, Kyritsis AP, Gleason MJ, et al. Treatment of recurrent malignant gliomas with high-dose 13-cis-retinoic acid. Clin Cancer Res 1996; 2(12):1931–5.

[41] Kaba SE, Langford LA, Yung WK, et al. Resolution of recurrent malignant ganglioglioma after treatment with cis-retinoic acid. J Neurooncol 1996; 30(1):55–60.

[42] DiGiovanna JJ, Patronas N, Katz D, et al. Xeroderma pigmentosum: spinal cord astrocytoma with 9-year survival after radiation and isotretinoin therapy. J Cutan Med Surg 1998;2(3):153–8.

[43] Strauss JS, Rapini RP, Shalita AR, et al. Isotretinoin therapy for acne: results of a multicenter dose-response study. J Am Acad Dermatol 1984;10(3):490–6.

[44] Stainforth JM, Layton AM, Taylor JP, et al. Isotretinoin for the treatment of acne vulgaris: which factors may predict the need for more than one course? Br J Dermatol 1993;129(3):297–301.

[45] Kus S. Vitamin E does not reduce the side-effects of isotretinoin in the treatment of acne vulgaris. Int J Dermatol 2005;44:248–51.

[46] Wysowski DK, Pitts M, Beitz J. Depression and suicide in patients treated with isotretinoin. N Engl J Med 2001;344(6):460.

[47] Marqueling AL, Zane LT. Depression and suicidal behavior in acne patients treated with isotretinoin: a systematic review. Semin Cutan Med Surg 2005; 24(2):92–102.

[48] Rappaport EB, Knapp M. Isotretinoin embryopathy—a continuing problem. J Clin Pharmacol 1989; 29(5):463–5.

[49] Lammer EJ, Chen DT, Hoar RM, et al. Retinoic acid embryopathy. N Engl J Med 1985;313(14): 837–41.

[50] Yu J, Gonzalez S, Martinez L, et al. Effects of retinoic acid on the neural crest-controlled organs of fetal rats. Pediatr Surg Int 2003;19(5):355–8.

[51] Pochi PE, Strauss JS. Sebaceous gland response in man to the administration of testosterone, delta-4-androstenedione, and dehydroisoandrosterone. J Invest Dermatol 1969;52(1):32–6.

[52] Thiboutot D, Harris G, Iles V, et al. Activity of the type 1 5 alpha-reductase exhibits regional differences in isolated sebaceous glands and whole skin. J Invest Dermatol 1995;105(2):209–14.

[53] Thiboutot D, Chen W. Update and future of hormonal therapy in acne. Dermatology 2003;206(1): 57–67.

[54] Thiboutot D, Gilliland K, Light J, et al. Androgen metabolism in sebaceous glands from subjects with and without acne. Arch Dermatol 1999;135(9): 1041–5.

[55] Shaw JC, White LE. Long-term safety of spironolactone in acne: results of an 8-year followup study. J Cutan Med Surg 2002;6(6):541–5.

[56] Yemisci A, Gorgulu A, Piskin S. Effects and side-effects of spironolactone therapy in women with acne. J Eur Acad Dermatol Venereol 2005;19(2):163–6.

[57] Tremblay MR, Luu-The V, Leblanc G, et al. Spironolactone-related inhibitors of type II 17beta-hydroxysteroid dehydrogenase: chemical synthesis, receptor binding affinities, and proliferative/antiproliferative activities. Bioorg Med Chem 1999;7(6): 1013–23.

[58] Zouboulis CC, Akamatsu H, Stephanek K, et al. Androgens affect the activity of human sebocytes in culture in a manner dependent on the localization of the sebaceous glands and their effect is antagonized by spironolactone. Skin Pharmacol 1994;7(1–2):33–40.

[59] Archer JS, Chang RJ. Hirsutism and acne in polycystic ovary syndrome. Best Pract Res Clin Obstet Gynaecol 2004;18(5):737–54.

[60] Harper JC. Antiandrogen therapy for skin and hair disease. Dermatol Clin 2006;24(2):137–43, v.

[61] Shaw JC. Low-dose adjunctive spironolactone in the treatment of acne in women: a retrospective analysis of 85 consecutively treated patients. J Am Acad Dermatol 2000;43(3):498–502.

[62] Hughes BR, Cunliffe WJ. Tolerance of spironolactone. Br J Dermatol 1988;118(5):687–91.

[63] Yamamoto A, Ito M. Topical spironolactone reduces sebum secretion rates in young adults. J Dermatol 1996;23(4):243–6.

[64] Lubbos HG, Hasinski S, Rose LI, et al. Adverse effects of spironolactone therapy in women with acne. Arch Dermatol 1998;134(9):1162–3.

[65] Haroun M. Hormonal therapy of acne. J Cutan Med Surg 2004;8(Suppl 4):6–10.

[66] Stewart ME, Greenwood R, Cunliffe WJ, et al. Effect of cyproterone acetate-ethinyl estradiol treatment on the proportions of linoleic and sebaleic acids in various skin surface lipid classes. Arch Dermatol Res 1986;278(6):481–5.

[67] Poulin Y. Practical approach to the hormonal treatment of acne. J Cutan Med Surg 2004;8(Suppl 4):16–21.

[68] Cunliffe WJ, Bottomley WW. Antiandrogens and acne. A topical approach? Arch Dermatol 1992; 128(9):1261–4.

[69] Huber J, Walch K. Treating acne with oral contraceptives: use of lower doses. Contraception 2006; 73(1):23–9.

[70] Dodin S, Faure N, Cedrin I, et al. Clinical efficacy and safety of low-dose flutamide alone and combined with an oral contraceptive for the treatment of idiopathic hirsutism. Clin Endocrinol (Oxf) 1995;43(5):575–82.

[71] Wysowski DK, Freiman JP, Tourtelot JB, et al. Fatal and nonfatal hepatotoxicity associated with flutamide. Ann Intern Med 1993;118(11):860–4.

[72] Garcia Cortes M, Andrade RJ, Lucena MI, et al. Flutamide-induced hepatotoxicity: report of a case series. Rev Esp Enferm Dig 2001;93(7):423–32.

[73] Muderris II, Bayram F, Guven M. Treatment of hirsutism with lowest-dose flutamide (62.5 mg/day). Gynecol Endocrinol 2000;14(1):38–41.

[74] Thornton MJ, Taylor AH, Mulligan K, et al. The distribution of estrogen receptor beta is distinct to that of estrogen receptor alpha and the androgen receptor in human skin and the pilosebaceous unit. J Investig Dermatol Symp Proc 2003;8(1):100–3.

[75] Pelletier G, Ren L. Localization of sex steroid receptors in human skin. Histol Histopathol 2004;19(2): 629–36.

[76] Hay JB, Hodgins MB, Donnelly JB. Human skin androgen metabolism and preliminary evidence for its control by two forms of 17 β-hydroxysteroid oxidoreductase. J Endocrinol 1982;93(3):403–13.

[77] Sawaya ME, Price VH. Different levels of 5α-reductase type I and II, aromatase, and androgen receptor in hair follicles of women and men with androgenetic alopecia. J Invest Dermatol 1997;109:296–300.

[78] Kariya Y, Moriya T, Suzuki T, et al. Sex steroid hormone receptors in human skin appendage and its neoplasms. Endocr J 2005;52(3):317–25.

[79] Thiboutot D. New treatments and therapeutic strategies for acne. Arch Fam Med 2000;9(2):179–87.

[80] Davies S, Dai D, Wolf DM, et al. Immunomodulatory and transcriptional effects of progesterone through progesterone A and B receptors in Hec50co poorly differentiated endometrial cancer cells. J Soc Gynecol Investig 2004;11(7):494–9.

[81] van Vloten WA, van Haselen CW, van Zuuren EJ, et al. The effect of 2 combined oral contraceptives containing either drospirenone or cyproterone acetate on acne and seborrhea. Cutis 2002;69(4 Suppl):2–15.

Dermatol Clin 25 (2007) 147–155

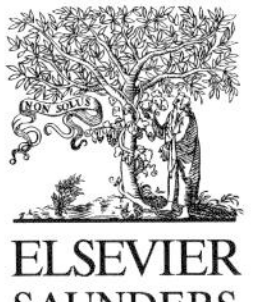

DERMATOLOGIC
CLINICS

Topical Immunomodulation: Modes of Action with Clinical Correlation

Neal Bhatia, MD

University of Wisconsin Medical School, 3119 S. Clement Avenue, Suite 100, Milwaukee, WI 53207, USA

The immune system affects almost every aspect of cutaneous biology. Abnormalities in immunosurveillance are involved in development and progression of inflammatory dermatoses, carcinogenesis and tumor genesis, and the consequence of cutaneous infections. In other words, most skin diseases, inflammatory or neoplastic, correlate with the immune system being "out of whack"—working too hard, not hard enough, lacking surveillance, or being dysregulated [1].

Several mechanisms result in cutaneous dysregulation and immunosuppression. Functional leukopenia within the skin occurs secondary to chronic photodamage, that is, years of ultraviolet A (UVA) and ultraviolet B (UVB) radiation causing depletion and stabilization of lymphocyte and mast cell populations. Iatrogenic sources of immune system abnormalities include chemotherapy and systemic immunosuppressants, such as corticosteroids, cyclosporin, tacrolimus, and azathioprine, all of which have significant impact on skin diseases. More importantly, there are a myriad of autoimmune diseases that involve different forms of hypersensitivity reactions to create cutaneous sequelae [2,3].

On the other hand, dermatologists use topical immunomodulators on a daily basis to either upregulate or down-regulate an immune response that impacts patient care. There are many forms of immunomodulators with various mechanisms of action to perform one of two goals: to stimulate the immune system to work harder to modify a disease process, or to slow down the activities of cellular and/or humoral immune mechanisms that are promoting the disease. Using topical immunomodulation to treat a tumor, inflammatory disease, or the consequence of a chronic disease process requires an understanding of the mechanism of action of the therapy as well as the cutaneous responses that the immune system generates [1].

Review of immune mechanisms

The immune responses of the skin favor either cellular or humoral mechanisms depending on the target antigens involved (Table 1) [1].

This division is the result of the actions of the reticuloendothelial system. The dendritic cells in the skin process antigens via toll-like receptors (TLRs) that result in initiation of cytokine release. The TLR lies on the dendritic cell membrane and surveys for antigen, for example of solid tumor or microbial origin. A simple analogy would be if the dendritic cell were the lighthouse of the immune system, the TLR would be the radar. It is the processing of this antigen that leads to the ultimate direction of the T-helper cell (CD4+ cell) guided by the secretion of interleukin 1 (IL-1). Recognition of viral or tumor antigens more often involves a cellular profile, labeled as Th1, as compared with bacterial antigen or an autoimmune type of stimulus that creates the Th2 profile. There are exceptions to the rule; however, for the most part this pattern is followed to delineate the type of anticipated host response [4,5].

For an antigen to be processed by the TLR, there is packaging in the cytoplasm by a protein called MyD88, which transfers the message to a nuclear transcription factor NF-κβ. NF-κβ is involved with many epidermal functions and modulates the metabolism of agents such as corticosteroid molecules by the DNA. After this

E-mail address: ndbhatia@juno.com

Table 1
Immune system functions

	Cellular	Humoral
Th responses	Th1	Th2
Primary cell	T cell	B cell
Antigens	Virus, Tumors	Bacteria
Cytokines	IL-2, IFNγ	IL-4, IL-5
Products	T-cell activation	Antibodies

Division of the immune mechanism based on the response to antigen with correlating T-helper cell profile, cytokines and cell lines.

Abbreviations: IFNγ, interferon gamma; IL, interleukin.

Data from Dahl MV. Clinical immunodermatology. 3rd edition. St. Louis (MO): Mosby; 1996.

step, there is translation of the RNA onto the ribosomes that direct the synthesis of the cytokines necessary for the immune response to be performed [4,5].

The secretion of cytokines by the appropriate cell line to activate another cell involves balance of the interactions (Table 2). As discussed in Table 1, there are feedback loops guided by the dendritic cells through the T-helper cells that modulate which effector lymphocytes, mast cells, neutrophils, or other cell lines become activated or proliferated [1].

What is an immunomodulator?

An agent that either stimulates or interferes with an immune response that is involved with pathogenesis can be considered an immunomodulator (Box 1).

Corticosteroids

Corticosteroids represent the complete immunosuppressant, having an impact on all levels of action including antigen presentation and activation of T cells, and an impact on effector processes such as release of prostaglandins and activity of neutrophils. These actions are what lead to rapid resolution of inflammation when administered topically, orally, and parenterally. The following are immunomodulation properties of corticosteroids [1]:

- ↓ IL-2, inhibiting T-cell activation
- ↓ Release of IL-1, IL-6, tumor necrosis factor (TNF)-α
- Blockade of prostaglandin synthesis
- ↓ Antigen processing
- Inhibition of neutrophil adhesion

Table 2
Cytokine functions: interleukins

IL-1	T-cell activation, ↑ IL-6	(Center)
IL-2	T-cell proliferation	(Quarterback)
IL-4	↑ IgE synthesis	(Running Back)
IL-5	↑ Eosinophils, B-cell activation	(Wide Receiver)
IL-6	NK cell activation	(Tight End)
IL-8	PMN activation and chemotaxis	(Kickoff Team)
IL-10	B-cell activation, ↑ Th-2 response	(Defense)
IL-12	↑ Th-1 response	(Coach)

An analogy of this sequence would be similar to football where the center (Langerhans' cell via IL-1) snaps the ball to the quarterback (T-helper cell via IL-2). From there the quarterback can hand the ball off to a running back (mast cell via IL-4), throw the ball to a wide receiver (eosinophil via IL-5), or throw to a tight end (NK cell via IL-6). This represents the progression from activation of the response, processing the target cells, and the performing of the response by effector cells. However, the game does not start without the kickoff, represented by the action of IL-8 on the neutrophil, which is often the first cell to be involved in an inflammatory cascade. The defense is represented by IL-10, which slows down the Th1 cellular response and promotes a humoral response by stimulating a Th2 profile. Finally, the coach is represented by IL-12, which by promoting the Th1 response serves to regulate the players on the field as well as up-regulating the activity of IL-1, analogous to sending in another play.

Abbreviations: Ig, immunoglobulin; IL, interleukin; NK, natural killer.

Data from Dahl MV. Clinical immunodermatology. 3rd edition. St. Louis (MO): Mosby; 1996.

However, when left unregulated this immunosuppression can lead to multiple consequences including infections, secondary malignancy, and alterations in fibrosis normally controlled by Th1-balanced cellular immunity [1].

For example, corticosteroids are the mainstay of treatment in eczematous dermatoses primarily because of their effect on IL-2. Once the activation of T cells is blocked, there is no secretion of IL-4 and IL-5 to stimulate mast cells and eosinophils, which are at high levels in early and late stages of atopic dermatitis, respectively. In addition, inhibition of the actions of prostaglandins favorably impacts pruritus, erythema from vasodilation, and other components of the disease other than inflammation [5].

An unfortunate consequence of overuse of corticosteroids, aside from the well-known sequelae of cutaneous atrophy and striae (Figs. 1

Box 1. A list of the more common immunomodulators used in dermatology

- Corticosteroids
- Calcineurin inhibitors
  Tacrolimus
  Pimecrolimus

- Imiquimod
- Calcipotriene
- Retinoids
- Topical chemotherapy
  5-FU
  Nitrogen mustard

- Antibiotics
  Tetracyclines

- Squaric acid
- Dapsone
- Nonsteroidal anti-inflammatory drugs (NSAIDs)
- Azelaic acid
- Antioxidants
  Green tea extract
  Cyclopamine

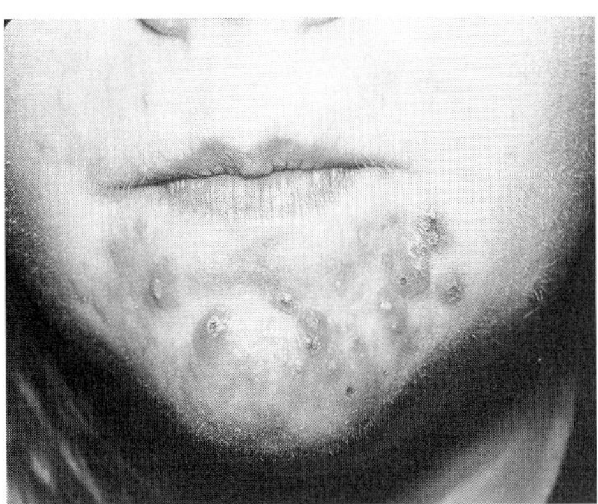

Fig. 2. Perioral dermatitis as a result of overuse of topical corticosteroids on the face.

and 2), is the induction of a "steroid addiction" [6]. This entity is often seen where there is a high suspicion from months to years of chronic eczematous diseases, when itch is out of proportion to the visible eruption, or where there has been prolonged use of combination products such as corticosteroid/antifungal preparations. Rebound

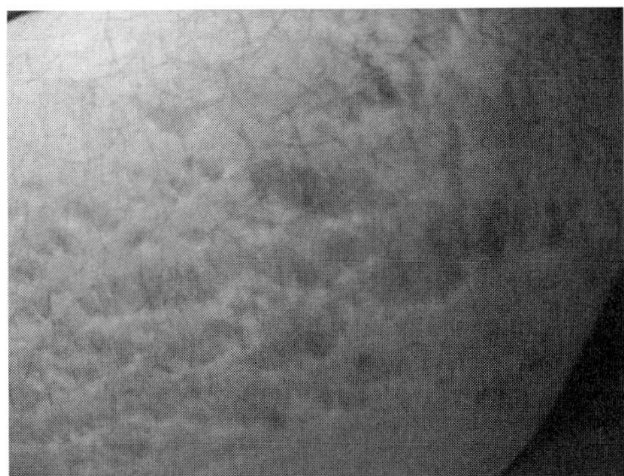

Fig. 1. Striae as a consequence of topical corticosteroid overuse.

vasodilation occurs after corticosteroid-induced vasoconstriction wanes. This often correlates to high serum levels of nitric oxide, which usually resolves after topical corticosteroid application is withdrawn; however, there is persistent elevation during flare and corticosteroid use. Addressing the history of overuse is the key to intervention, and treatment starts with introducing nonsteroid alternatives such as topical lidocaine or pramoxine for treatment of itch where the eruption has resolved [6].

Bacterial superantigens may have some influences on the mechanisms of corticosteroid resistance. For example, the superantigen protein A on *Staphylococcus aureus* binds to lymphocytes and, via transcription factor of corticosteroid-sensitive genes, creates a shift in the expression of steroid receptors from an alpha form to beta form, which is over 100 times less potent for steroid binding. The end result is a functional insensitivity to corticosteroids that necessitates more frequent application to create the same immunosuppressive effect, exposing the treated skin to more potential adverse consequences of therapy. As a result, this concept suggests a therapeutic benefit related to use of antibimicrobial agents to alter the population of *S aureus*, thus reducing this potential alteration in steroid receptor expression [7].

Calcineurin inhibitors

Calcineurin inhibitors (CIs) are viable alternatives as components of many treatment regimens once dominated by corticosteroids. This is primarily because of their actions as cell-selective inhibitors of inflammatory cytokines in T cells and mast cells while there appears to be no effect on keratinocytes, fibroblasts, endothelial cells, or Langerhans' cells. Advantages of lymphocyte selectivity include intact tumor surveillance; recognition of antigen on bacteria, viruses, and dermatophytes; and activity against mechanisms for pruritus and inflammation without affecting overall immunity status. More importantly, by avoiding depletion of Langerhans' cells from the epidermis, induction of skin atrophy, striae, and telangiectasia, as well as HPA-axis suppression, these drugs can be used safely for longer periods thus making shorter bursts of higher potency topical corticosteroids more effective [8–10].

CIs bind to binding factors or immunophilins (CIBP) in the cytoplasm. For cyclosporin, the immunophilin is cyclophilin, whereas tacrolimus and pimecrolimus bind to macrophilin 12, formerly known as FK506-binding protein (FK-BP) [8–10]. The following are the immunomodulatory effects of the calcineurin inhibitors tacrolimus and pimecrolimus [11]:

- ↓ IL-2, inhibiting T-cell activation
- ↓ IL-4, IL-13, and other cytokines
- ↓ Inflammatory mediator release from skin mast cells and basophils
- ↓ Expression FcεRI
- ↓ Dendritic cell presentation of antigen to autologous lymphocytes

Once bound together, the inhibitor/immunophilin (CI/CIBP) complex blocks the calcium-dependent serine-threonine phosphatase, calcineurin. This, in turn, prevents calcineurin from causing dephosphorylation of specific cytoplasmic proteins known as nuclear factors of activated T cells (NF-AT). The proteins are then prevented from translocating into the nucleus where they would normally bind to the promoter region of the gene to up-regulate transcription of genes that code for inflammatory cytokines. In some instances, NF-AT interacts with other nuclear subunits/factors (ie, AP-1) to then exert the same effect in gene transcription. Thus, inhibitors of calcineurin inhibit NF-AT–dependent gene transcription and IL-2, IL-4, and IL-5 transcription, thereby blocking T-cell activation and proliferation [11–13].

This class of drugs has recently drawn attention from the Food and Drug Administration over concerns of potential carcinogenesis based on laboratory data in animal models, suggesting the production of lymphomas. However, tested subjects were exposed to over 30 times the oral dosage normally administered, as opposed to topical therapy used for treatment of patients. In addition, based on the premise that cutaneous dendritic cells are not affected by the topical application of these macrolide derivatives, it could be concluded that antigen processing tumor surveillance by the reticuloendothelial system would not be compromised at the standard topical doses. Finally, the subtypes of lymphomas that have been rarely reported in subjects using topical CIs do not correlate with those known to occur in patients undergoing prolonged systemic immunosuppression because of underlying conditions such as organ transplantation. This raises significant uncertainty regarding the potential for carcinogenesis in patients appropriately treated with topical CIs [9,14].

Vitamin D analogs

Many derivatives of vitamin D and their releasing hormones such as calcitriol have immunomodulator effects. There are vitamin D receptors found on important cell lines such as dermal fibroblasts, T and B lymphocytes, monocytes, and macrophages. These agents interact with high-affinity nuclear receptors to regulate gene expression. For example, calcitriol regulates transcription through ligand-dependent inhibition of activator protein-1, NF-AT, and NF-κβ. The resultant effects are a decrease in levels of IL-2, IL-6, IL-8, interferon gamma (IFNγ), and granulocyte macrophage colony-stimulating factor (GM-CSF). In addition, vitamin D analogs have been shown to increase IL-10 production in psoriatic lesions and decrease IL-6 and IL-8 secretion by keratinocytes. This observation suggests a reduction in cellular immunity because of reduction in the circulating levels of functional lymphocytes and neutrophils. Topical preparations such as calcipotriene display less potent immune effects. The primary outcomes in conditions such as psoriasis and morphea, where calcipotriene is often part of the regimen include (1) dephosphorylation and deactivation of epidermal growth factor, (2) inhibition of proliferation of keratinocytes, and (3) stimulation of terminal differentiation [15,16].

The activity of vitamin D analogs on receptors is mediated through both up-regulation and down-regulation. Although the exact mechanism of down-regulation is unclear, it appears to be accomplished by either binding to negative receptor elements in the promoter section of genes or by antagonizing the action of/competing with certain transcription factors such as AP-1. Following is a list of the effects of vitamin D analogs on leukocytes [15,16]:

- Inhibition of T-cell proliferation
- Induction of hypo-responsiveness to allo- and self-antigens
- Inhibition of IL-2 and IFNγ production
- Inhibition of Th1 cell development
- Variable effects on IL-4 production
- Increased production of IL-10
- Increased expression of CD152
- Down-regulation of CD95 expression
- Enhanced frequency of regulatory T cells

Retinoids

Retinoid molecules serve as immunomodulators via several mechanisms. Their impact on cytokine production begins from the binding to retinoic acid receptors (RARs) in the cell nucleus. Once bound, the RAR/retinoid complex down-regulates the expression of other genes by antagonizing or competing with transcription factors such as AP-1. The exact mechanism of this interaction, often called "transcriptional crosstalk," is yet to be elucidated [17,18].

Retinoids exhibit anti-inflammatory properties via inhibition of the expression of inflammation-associated proteins, including HLA-DR and adhesion molecules on lymphocytes. Another example is the reduction in circulating levels of IL-6 in skin treated with retinoids, specifically seen in lesions of Kaposi's sarcoma treated with alitretinoin. These represent situations where the induction of immunoglobulin production in B lymphocytes and proliferation and differentiation of T lymphocytes into cytotoxic cells are all affected in an immune process [18–20].

Finally, retinoids inhibit expression of toll-like receptor 2 (TLR-2), which results in reduction in cellular inflammation mechanisms. In acne vulgaris, *P acnes* stimulates immune responses via its binding activity to TLR-2 on keratinocytes resulting in the release of IL-1 alpha. This appears to initiate inflammatory cascades that lead to higher populations of CD4+ and CD8+ lymphocytes in acne papules. The following lists the impact of *P acnes* on inflammation [21–23]:

- Releases chemotactic factors to attract polymorphonuclear cells, monocytes, and lymphocytes
  - MIP-1 alpha and beta, MCP-1 (macrophages)

  - IL-8 (PMN attractant)
  - ITAC, TNF

- Activates complement cascade
- Produces free fatty acid from metabolism of triglycerides in sebum-releasing hydrolytic enzymes that may release the content of the follicle
  - Stimulates TLR-2 expression

Azelaic acid

There are many properties of azelaic acid that make it an immunomodulator. In the treatment of acne and rosacea, azelaic acid preparations demonstrate anti-inflammatory activity via effects on neutrophils and oxygen free radicals. Azelaic acid also impacts melanogenesis by inhibiting the effects of tyrosinase [24,25]. The following is a list of the immunomodulator effects of azelaic acid [24]:

- Inhibits tyrosinase
- Acts as a free radical scavenger in vitro
- Inhibits oxy-radical toxicity to neutrophils
- Diminishes potency of inflammation via reduction of reactive oxygen species

"Nonspecific" immunotherapeutic agents

Dinitrochlorobenzene (DNCB) and squaric acid dibutylester (SADBE) represent two contact sensitizing agents that stimulate immune reactions. The mechanism of SADBE likely involves the generation of a delayed-type (cell-mediated) hypersensitivity reaction at the site of the verruca, requiring antigen presentation to CD4+ cells. In addition, there appears to be recruitment of CD8+ cells and an overall up-regulation of Th1 responses. The result of this is demonstrated in conditions where cellular immunity is essential to control of the disease process. For example, in warts there is induction of cytotoxic lymphocyte killing of virally infected cells [26].

Immunotherapies may work by acting as haptens, complexing with viral antigens and thereby inducing a papillomavirus-specific antigen presentation and immune response. However, as opposed to a tumor, an immune "process" that creates a dermatosis such as atopic dermatitis that is primarily a Th2 disease can be modified or converted to reflect a more cellular profile. This has been demonstrated by Mills and colleagues [27] where squaric acid was used to treat eczematous plaques. Weekly patch application for 12 to

18 hours took place with initial sensitization with 1.5 mg, then 0.5 mg per week for the treatment duration. The results of their study demonstrated 7 of 9 patients had more than 50% reduction in body surface area (BSA) involved. More importantly, there were no major changes in serum IL-2, NK cells, or other T-cell markers.

Candida antigen is also an immunomodulator extract that is used to treat verruca by intralesional injuction. This form of therapy induces expression of TLR-2, TLR-8, and TLR-9. This results in enhanced processing of viral antigens where the host immunity is often insufficient to recognize and eradicate the wart [28].

Polyphenon

Polyphenon(R) E ointment contains catechines that have immunostimulatory properties that counteract specific changes in tumor cells. Many of the actions are based on the antioxidant properties leading to procytokine release, although the true mechanisms are not clear. Early clinical phase II trials over 4 months for actinic keratoses (AKs) have revealed reduction of visible skin lesions and demonstration of subclinical disease. In addition, clinical phase III trials for condyloma studying more than 1000 patients showed the significant efficacy and high safety of polyphenon(R) E ointment [29,30]. Immunomodulators that contain or that are derived from green tea extract, which is steamed and dried out of plants, often need butylated hydroxytoluene for stability. The antioxidant effects protect against UV resulting in reduced UV-induced edema and erythema as well as reduced formation of thymidine-thymidine (T-T) dimmers. The result of this is less DNA mutagenesis and photocarcinogenesis [30,31].

Imiquimod

Imiquimod is a member of the imidazoquinolinamine family. The mechanism of action of imiquimod classifies it as an immune response modifier, based on the augmentation of cellular immune responses and recruitment of cytokines and natural killer cell activity. The main impact is up-regulation of the primary Th-1 cytokines IL-1, IL-6, IL-8, IL-12, IFNα, and TNF-α. However, there are no effects on IL-2, which signifies that imiquimod does not create a new immune process; rather, it augments a response that is already active to make it more effective. In addition, there is inhibition of the Th-2 response, resulting in

diminished levels of IL-4 and IL-5. Therefore, imiquimod is useful in disease states requiring cellular immunity such as tumors and viral infections, as well as conditions of Th-2 overexpression like atopic or autoimmune states [4,5].

The concept of augmenting an immune response and promoting cellular immunity is the basis for modifying the process of the disease, not just alleviating symptoms. For example, this is important for preventing long-term outcomes such as invasive squamous cell carcinoma occurring in skin that is affected by extensive photodamage or multiple AKs. This is based on the idea that antigen processing leads to inflammation that is focused against that target, whether it is inflammatory, infectious, or neoplastic. When an inflammatory response is directed in this fashion with a purpose, it can be considered to be a primary component of the process to modify the disease. The opposite effect will be where inflammation is recruited as an aftereffect of the disease or treatment, but has no impact on the progression or future of the disease. In this case, the inflammation is a reaction rather than a response and is a secondary phenomenon [4,5]. An example of this latter scenario is the inflammatory reaction that occurs after application of 5-fluorouracil to skin affected by AKs (Table 3).

The clinical signs of immune stimulation can vary among patients in that responses may range from minimal erythema to aggressive crusted plaques around the application sites ("brisk response"). Some patients treated with topical imiquimod do not demonstrate erythema or induration at the site of application yet when assessed at the end point of treatment there is clinical evidence of efficacy, for example with reduction in size of tumors or warts or numbers of AKs. This may be explained by a study done by Li and colleagues [32] where a randomized group of patients was treated with different dosage

Table 3
Mechanisms of action: imiquimod versus 5-fluorouracil

Imiquimod	5-Fluorouracil
Immune recruitment	Keratinization repair
Dermal effects	Epidermal effects
■ Induration	■ Heavy crust
■ Erythema	■ Desquamation
	■ Moderate Itch + Pain
Memory induction	Local effects
Inflammation as primary outcome	Inflammation as secondary outcome

protocols up to the point of erythema but did not actually become red. However, there was improvement overall in the conditions treated, which suggested that individual patients have a biweekly, every other day, every day, twice a day, and so forth response profile. The message to consider is that the suberythema effects correlate to recruitment of cytokines, not to clinical inflammation. Therefore, patients may not demonstrate a clinically visible inflammatory response even though their immune system has processed the antigens involved and the directed inflammatory cascade is augmented. Clinically, it is clear that patients need to continue the course to the end point of treatment even if there is no evidence of erythema. On the other hand, the patients who experience vigorous reactions may often have concomitant superinfections in the treatment sites. This is often because of photodamaged skin having lost its baseline immune surveillance resulting in colonization of gram-positive and anaerobic skin organisms such as *S aureus* or *S epidermidis* species. Isolation of *S aureus* can result in aggressive reactions in eroded lesions resulting in heavy crust and erosions, whether it is a function of infection versus colonization and is often secondary to the augmented immune response. One possibility is a result of the activity of protein A superantigen from *S aureus* [7]. Another possible explanation is enhanced CD8+ recruitment to the site of application because more than one TLR has been stimulated to recognize bacterial antigens, such as TLR-2 (bacterial peptidoglycan) or TLR-4 (bacterial lipopolysaccharide) (Figs. 3–5) [22].

Miscellaneous immunomodulators

Many preparations exist that have immunomodulatory properties to varying degrees and strengths (Box 2). Botanical extracts have multiple effects on the immune system depending on their mechanisms of action. Allantoin is derived from oxidation of uric acid and is found in plants, although other purified sources are typically found for use on skin. The resultant mechanisms of action of application include promotion of photodamage repair, induction of cell proliferation, and reduction of UV-induced inflammation [33].

Aloe vera is an established wound-healing preparation that must have at least 10% aloe vera to demonstrate any observable benefit. It is composed of 99.5% water and 0.05% plant-derived active ingredient in a mixture of mucopolysaccharides, amino acids, and minerals. It is

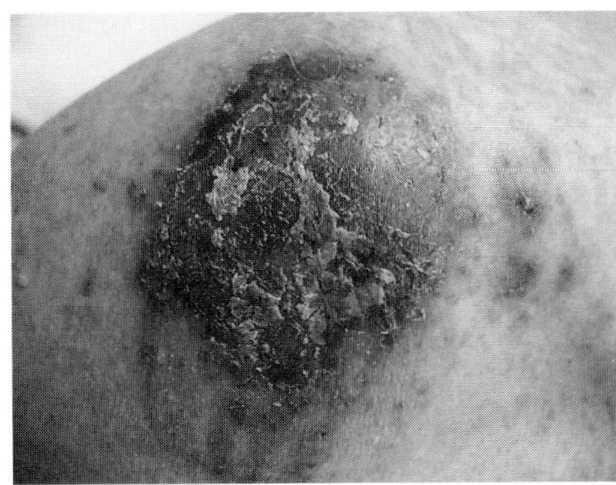

Fig. 3. Patient on imiquimod therapy for superficial basal cell carcinoma with a brisk reaction at 4 weeks into treatment. This patient could be treated with a topical antibiotic to reduce the severity of the response if is symptomatic, but the course of imiquimod is best continued to keep the augmented immune response at a high level.

often prepared as either a colorless gel or in a powder form in skin care products. *Gingko biloba* is an antioxidant extract that contains polyphenols, flavonoids, and flavonol glycosides. Its immunomodulatory effects take place on collagen and stroma via stimulation of fibroblast proliferation and extracellular fibronectin [31].

Finally, the spice curcumin, an ingredient in common turmeric or curry powder spice and integral in the preparation of Indian and other Asian foods, has been observed to have antitumor and anti-inflammatory properties. It has been prepared for investigations in a variety of vehicles,

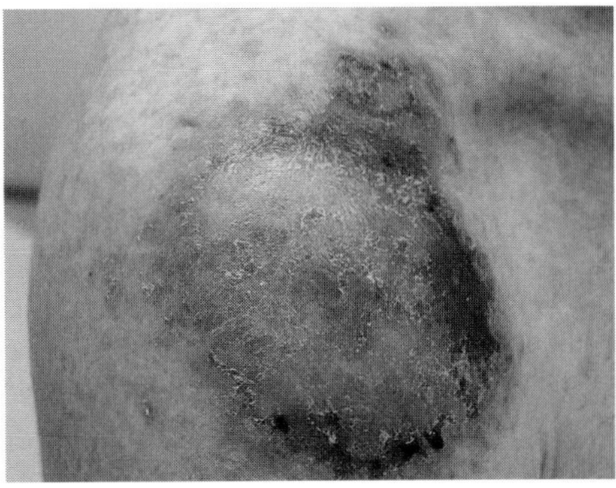

Fig. 4. At 8 weeks into the course of daily treatment with imiquimod, the inflammatory response begins to subside. This is a marker that the tumor burden and its associated antigenic stimulus is decreasing. As a result there is less tumor antigen available for the immune system to process. It is at this stage where frequency of dosing could be decreased.

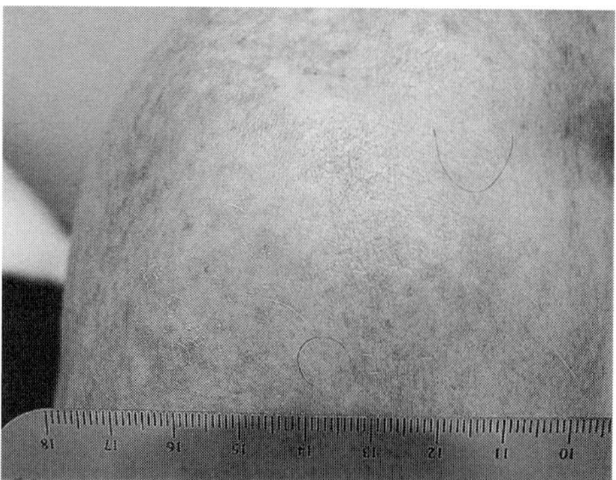

Fig. 5. The same patient 6 months after completion of treatment has no visible residual tumor.

including oral capsules, topicals, and intravenous and subcutaneous injections. Clinical trials testing its effects on melanoma, colon cancer, pancreatic cancer, multiple myeloma, and breast cancer are under way. Its mechanisms of action are based on the suppression of nuclear factor-kappa β (NF-κβ) binding activity and upstream regulator I-kappa β -alpha kinase (IKK). Spices that appear to block NF-κβ include the following [30,34]:

Box 2. Other topical "immunomodulators"

Skin Zinc© –zinc pyrithione
- antifungal and antibacterial ingredient

Freederm© 1% hydrocortisone
Eczana© tea tree oil
- antiseptic, a fungicide, and a mild solvent.

Oenothein-B©
- antiviral, antitumor, and antihyperandrogenic applications.

Canadian willow herb extract
- nonsteroidal anti-inflammatory activity
- skin cleansers, fresheners, and soothers

Oregon grape extract

Data from Glaser DA. Sorting through the claims of topical botanical anti-inflammatory agents. Practical Dermatology 2005;2:16–8.

- Curcumin
- Red pepper (capsaicin)
- Cloves
- Ginger
- Basil
- Rosemary

Once down-regulated by curcumin, there was reduction of tumor proliferation and induction of apoptosis [30,34]. The following are the immuno-modulatory mechanisms of curcumin:

- Suppression of NF-κβ
- NF-κβ binding activity and upstream regular IKK were down-regulated by curcumin, which also induced apoptosis
- Influence of IL-6 to allow for Akt phosphorylation instead of suppressing it
- Activation of capsase-8
- Increase in p53 activity

Summary

Many classes and preparations of immunomodulators are available to the clinician, serving either as a stimulatory or an inhibitory influence on a variety of disease states. To maximize their efficacy, it is important for the clinician to take a step back from the usual routine of treating symptoms and consider the immune processes that took place to create inflammation, tumors, or responses to infections. From there, after considering both the short-term and long-term consequences of the treatment, one can match the immune profile of the disease to that of the treatment. Most importantly, immunomodulators provide the opportunity to do what is best for the patient at that time as well as for control of the future of the disease, whether it is acute or chronic.

Acknowledgment

All photographs are of patients seen by Neal Bhatia, MD. The photographs are used with the patients' written consent.

References

[1] Dahl MV. Clinical immunodermatology. 3rd edition. St. Louis (MO): Mosby; 1996.
[2] Kang K, Stevens S, Cooper K. Pathophysiology of ultraviolet irradiation. Available at: http://www.aad.org/professionals/Residents/MedStudCoreCurr/DCUVIrradiation.htm. Accessed June 15, 2005.

[3] Ullrich SE. Mechanisms underlying UV-induced immune suppression. Mutat Res 2005;571:185–205.

[4] Miller Rl, Gerster JF, Owens ML, et al. Imiquimod applied topically: a novel immune response modifier and a new class of drug. Int J Immunopharmacol 1999;21:1–14.

[5] Suzuki H, Wang B, Amerio P, et al. Imiquimod, a novel topical immune response modifier induces migration of Langerhans' cells. J Invest Dermatol 1999;112(4):628.

[6] Rapaport M. Anecdotal as printed in Dermatology Times, Jan 1, 2004. Arch Dermatol, in press.

[7] Nelson HS, Leung DYM, Bloom JW. Update on glucocorticoid action and resistance. J Allergy Clin Immunol 2003;111(1):3–22.

[8] Grassberger M, Baumruker T, Enz A, et al. A novel anti-inflammatory drug, SDZ ASM 981, for the treatment of skin diseases: in vitro pharmacology. Br J Dermatol 1999;141:264–73.

[9] Eichenfield LF, Lucky AW, Boguniewicz M, et al. Safety and efficacy of pimecrolimus (ASM 981) cream 1% in the treatment of mild and moderate atopic dermatitis in children and adolescents. J Am Acad Dermatol 2002;46:495–504.

[10] Hutch T, Kapp A, Spergel J. Immunomodulation and safety of topical calcineurin inhibitors for the treatment of atopic dermatitis. Dermatology 2005; 211:174–87.

[11] Marsland AM, Griffiths CE. The macrolide immunosuppressants in dermatology: mechanisms of action. Eur J Dermatol 2002;12:618–22.

[12] Russell JJ. Topical tacrolimus: a new therapy for atopic dermatitis. Am Fam Physician 2002;66: 1899–902.

[13] Bornhövd E, Burgdorf WH, Wollenberg A. Macrolactam immunomodulators for topical treatment of inflammatory skin diseases. J Am Acad Dermatol 2001;45:736–43.

[14] Meurer M, Fölster-Holst R, Wozel G, et al, for the CASM-DE-01 Study Group. Pimecrolimus cream in the long-term management of atopic dermatitis in adults: a six-month study. Dermatology 2002; 205:271–7.

[15] Adorini L. Immunomodulatory effects of vitamin D receptor ligands in autoimmune diseases. Int Immunopharmacol 2002;2:1017–28.

[16] Nagpal S, Lu J, Boehm MF. Vitamin D analogs: mechanism of action and therapeutic applications. Curr Med Chem 2001;8:1661–79.

[17] Duvic M, Nagpal S, Asano AT, et al. Molecular mechanisms of tazarotene action in psoriasis. J Am Acad Dermatol 1997;37:S18–24.

[18] Nagpal S, Athanikar J, Chandraratna RA. Separation of transactivation and AP1 antagonism functions of retinoic acid receptor alpha. J Biol Chem 1995;270:923–7.

[19] Zouboulis CC. Retinoids—which dermatological indications will benefit in the near future? Skin Pharmacol Appl Skin Physiol 2001;14:303–15.

[20] Saurat JH. Retinoids and psoriasis: novel issues in retinoid pharmacology and implications for psoriasis treatment. J Am Acad Dermatol 1999;41:S2–6.

[21] McInturff JE. The role of toll-like receptors in the pathophysiology of acne. Semin Cutan Med Surg 2005;24:73–8.

[22] Kang SSW, Kauls LS, Gaspari AA. Toll-like receptors: applications to dermatologic disease. J Am Acad Dermatol 2006;54(6):951–83.

[23] Millikan L. The rationale for using a topical retinoid for inflammatory acne. Am J Clin Dermatol 2003; 4(2):75–80.

[24] Thiboutot D, Thieroff-Ekerdt R, Graupe K. Efficacy and safety of azelaic acid (15%) gel as a new treatment for papulopustular rosacea: results from two vehicle-controlled, randomized phase III studies. J Am Acad Dermatol 2003;48(6):836–45.

[25] Schallreuter KU, Wood JW. A possible mechanism of action for azelaic acid in the human epidermis. Arch Dermatol Res 1990;282(3):168–71.

[26] Silverberg NB, Lim JK, Paller AS, et al. Squaric acid immunotherapy for warts in children. J Am Acad Dermatol 2000;42(5):803–8.

[27] Mills LB, Mordan LJ, Roth HL, et al. Treatment of severe atopic dermatitis by topical immune modulation using dinitrochlorobenzene. J Am Acad Dermatol 2000;42:687–9.

[28] Signore RJ, et al. Candida immunotherapy of warts. Arch Dermatol 2001;137:1250–1.

[29] Chow HH. Pharmacokinetics and safety of green tea polyphenols after multiple-dose administration of epigallocatechin gallate and Polyphenon E in healthy individuals. Clin Cancer Res 2003;9:3312–9.

[30] Wright T, Spencer J, Flowers F. Chemoprevention of nonmelanoma skin cancer. J Am Acad Dermatol 2006;54:933–46.

[31] Glaser DA. Sorting through the claims of topical botanical anti-inflammatory agents. Practical Dermatology 2005;17–8.

[32] Li V, et al. Poster Presented at the AAD 2005 Annual Meeting. 2005.

[33] Strickland FM. Immune protection, natural products, and skin cancer: is there anything new under the sun? J Drugs Dermatol 2006;512–17.

[34] Aggarwal B. Dermatology Times. September 1, 2005.

DERMATOLOGIC CLINICS

Dermatol Clin 25 (2007) 157–164

Methicillin-Sensitive and Methicillin-Resistant *Staphylococcus aureus*: Management Principles and Selection of Antibiotic Therapy

Dirk M. Elston, MD[a,b,*]

[a]*Department of Dermatology, Geisinger Medical Center, 100 North Academy Ave., Danville, PA 17822, USA*
[b]*Department of Pathology, Geisinger Medical Center, 100 North Academy Ave., Danville, PA 17822, USA*

Highly virulent community-acquired Methicillin-resistant *Staphylococcus aureus* (CA-MRSA) was first reported in Australia in 1993 [1]. More recently, CA-MRSA strains have been reported in many locations across North America, Europe, and Asia. CA-MRSA strains tend to infect young and previously healthy individuals, especially athletes. Other groups at risk include military personnel, prison inmates, homosexuals, intravenous drug users, the homeless, Alaskan Natives, Native Americans, Pacific Islanders, and children in daycare [2–5]. Roughly three quarters of CA-MRSA infections present in the skin, with a typical presentation being a furuncle that rapidly evolves to an abscess [6–11].

Most CA-MRSA isolates have been associated with the type IV staphylococcal chromosomal cassette mec (SCCmec) coding for methicillin resistance, and the Panton-Valentine leukocidin (PVL) virulence factor [12]. CA-MRSA outbreaks have been reported in many locations in North America, but individual outbreaks may be restricted to small geographic areas. During an outbreak of 182 cases of CA-MRSA infection in Massachusetts, 27 of 33 patients (81%) were from a single town, and many lived within a single 1.96-km² area [13].

Increased prevalence of methicillin-resistant *Staphylococcus aureus* infections

A study of 2154 inpatient and outpatient MRSA isolates in San Francisco over a 7-year period showed a greater than fourfold increase in methicillin resistance between 1998 and 2002. Emergency department data from Oakland, California, indicate that CA-MRSA is now present in 51% of cultured skin and soft tissue infections [11]. In a South Texas children's hospital, 1002 MRSA cases were identified between 1990 and 2003, of which 928 (93%) were community acquired [14]. CA-MRSA has been noted in rural communities in Wisconsin and Alaska, as well as in such urban settings as Los Angeles and New York [15–17]. A recent study at a Rhode Island microbiology laboratory showed that 40% of MRSA isolates were CA-MRSA [18].

Predictably, community-associated strains have not remained isolated to the community, but have spread into health care settings. CA-MRSA strains have caused nosocomial prosthetic joint infections, and hospital transmission of CA-MRSA has been described in postpartum women with skin and soft tissue infections [19–21]. CA-MRSA transmission has also been reported in a neonatal intensive care unit [22]. A meta-analysis of retrospective studies published through 2003 found a CA-MRSA prevalence of 30.2% among hospital MRSA infections [23]. New names may have to be devised for "community-acquired" and "health care-associated" strains, as CA-MRSA strains have clearly crossed from the community into health care settings [24].

The author has been a consultant and speaker for Abbott Laboratories and Medicis Pharmaceuticals.

* Department of Dermatology, Geisinger Medical Center, 100 North Academy Ave., Danville, PA 17821.

E-mail address: delston@geisinger.edu

Virulence factors

CA-MRSA carrying the PVL virulence factor has proved to be highly virulent and well adapted to spread within communities. In an Alaskan study, PVL genes were present in 97% of CA-MRSA isolates but in no methicillin-susceptible isolates [25]. A study of patients receiving surgical treatment at an outpatient clinic in the San Francisco Bay area showed that 69% of the strains carried PVL [9].

Colonization and spread of methicillin-resistant *Staphylococcus aureus*

A retrospective cohort study suggested that contacts of CA-MRSA–colonized patients have a 7.5 times greater risk of colonization [26]. Those who are colonized commonly progress to develop a clinical infection over time [27].

Potential severity of methicillin-resistant *Staphylococcus aureus* infections

In a study of 57 pregnant women with CA-MRSA skin infection, 63% required hospital admission [28]. In a study of emergency department patients in Oakland, California, 26% of patients required admission [11]. Life-threatening skin infections, including necrotizing fasciitis, have been reported [29]. However most fatal CA-MRSA infections have presented with lung involvement rather than skin involvement. Forty-seven of 70 children with invasive CA-MRSA infections admitted to Texas Children's Hospital in Houston between August 1, 2001, and June 30, 2004, had abnormal pulmonary imaging findings. In comparison, only 12 of 43 patients admitted with community-acquired methicillin-susceptible *S aureus* (MSSA) infection had pulmonary symptoms [30]. Twelve adolescents with CA-MRSA infection were admitted to the Texas Children's Hospital pediatric intensive care unit with sepsis and coagulopathy between August 2002 and January 2004. Thirteen of the patients had pulmonary involvement or bone and joint infection. Ten patients had two or more bones or joints infected, and 3 of the patients died [31]. Fortunately, the CA-MRSA–associated pulmonary syndrome accounts for the minority of infections and few of these patients present with skin involvement.

Management of methicillin-resistant *Staphylococcus aureus* infections

The treatment for a cutaneous abscess remains drainage, whether or not the abscess is caused by MRSA. Laboratory-based sentinel surveillance data from Baltimore, Atlanta, and Minnesota collected between 2001 and 2002 revealed 1647 cases of CA-MRSA infection. Seventy-seven percent of infections presented as skin or soft tissue infection, and only 6% of patients had invasive disease. The organism was resistant to the prescribed antimicrobial agent in 73% of the reported cases, yet therapy to which the strain was resistant was not associated with adverse patient-reported outcomes if the abscess was incised and drained [32]. Other data also suggest that drainage alone may be adequate treatment for many MRSA abscesses. A review of 695 *S aureus* infections treated at the San Francisco General Hospital Integrated Soft Tissue Infection Clinic between July 1, 2000, and June 30, 2003, revealed that 76% of the isolates were MRSA. Thirty percent of the patients received a beta-lactam antibiotic inactive against MRSA, yet all had full resolution of their infection. The investigators suggested that antibiotic therapy directed at MRSA may not be needed in a large number of patients with soft tissue infections if drainage is performed [33]. In another study of 69 children with culture-proved CA-MRSA abscesses, drainage was performed in 96% of patients. Only 5 patients (7%) were initially prescribed an antibiotic to which their isolate was susceptible. Initial ineffective antibiotic therapy was not a statistically significant predictor of admission ($P = 1.0$). In contrast, lesion diameter >5 cm was a statistically significant predictor of hospitalization ($P = .0040$). Overall, there were no significant differences in response in the patients who never received an effective antibiotic compared with those who did. The authors of the study concluded that incision and drainage alone was effective management of CA-MRSA abscesses smaller than 5 cm in immunocompetent children [34]. The above evidence suggests that drainage alone may be effective therapy for many CA-MRSA abscesses. Failure to drain CA-MRSA abscesses may result in bad outcomes, even if effective antibiotic therapy is prescribed. In one case, bilateral blindness resulted from orbital cellulitis caused by CA-MRSA. Effective antibiotic therapy had been administered, but drainage was delayed [35].

Methicillin-resistant *Staphylococcus aureus* isolates and antibiotic resistance

In all MRSA isolates, the methicillin resistance gene is carried on the SCCmec. The type II cassette is common among HA-MRSA strains and codes for resistance to multiple antibiotics. HA-MRSA isolates with intermediate and full resistance to vancomycin and isolates resistant to newer drugs, such as linezolid, are particularly problematic [36]. SCCmec type IV is typically present in CA-MRSA strains. The gene cassette is quite small and codes only for methicillin resistance. Therefore CA-MRSA isolates are usually susceptible to a number of non–beta-lactam antibiotics.

Some CA-MRSA isolates have emerged that are resistant to multiple antibiotics. In 2004, a multiple-drug–resistant SCCmec IV CA-MRSA strain was isolated from a Japanese athlete presenting with an abscess. The strain expressed PVL, but also had a transmissible, multiple-drug–resistance plasmid [37]. Some isolates from Taipei carry a distinct SCCmec cassette designated type VT. These strains express PVL, but are resistant to multiple antibiotics [38]. In a study from a Taiwanese children's hospital, MRSA accounted for 47% of 114 community-acquired infections. Type IV SCCmec was only carried by 25% of the CA-MRSA isolates. Ninety-three percent of the CA-MRSA isolates demonstrated resistance to clindamycin, although 91% remained susceptible to trimethoprim–sulfamethoxazole. Many patients with CA-MRSA abscesses will resolve after drainage regardless of the susceptibility pattern. In this study, all superficial CA-MRSA soft tissue infections resolved without sequelae, even though 63% of the children were treated with antibiotics to which the organism was not susceptible [39].

Antibiotic therapy for methicillin-resistant *Staphylococcus aureus* infection

While drainage alone cures many CA-MRSA abscesses, some patients need antibiotic therapy. Sulfonamides remain the most valuable class of antibiotic for the treatment of CA-MRSA infections. Some concern has been raised about the possibility of sulfonamide resistance in areas with large HIV-positive populations because of the use of such agents as trimethoprim–sulfamethoxazole for pneumocystis prophylaxis. Although this remains a valid concern, one study found 100% of CA-MRSA isolates in the Oakland, California,

area to be susceptible to trimethoprim–sulfamethoxazole [5].

Although sulfonamide drugs generally remain a reliable choice for CA-MRSA infection requiring antibiotic treatment, and tetracyclines remain good alternative agents in most areas, lincosamide resistance is more problematic [40]. Clindamycin has been used successfully to treat a variety of CA-MRSA infections, including soft tissue infections, pneumonia, and musculoskeletal infections, but good outcome in many abscesses may be related to drainage rather than the antibiotic. The possibility of inducible clindamycin resistance has discouraged some physicians from prescribing clindamycin [41–44]. The inducible macrolide-lincosamide-streptogramin B phenotype is related to the erm gene. Strains with inducible resistance will test clindamycin-susceptible in vitro, but are erythromycin-resistant. If inducible resistance is present, there is a potential for treatment failure with clindamycin, despite the culture and sensitivity report indicating susceptibility. For this reason, some microbiology laboratories no longer report erythromycin-resistant staphylococci as sensitive to clindamycin. Rather, they issue a report stating that macrolide resistance may be a marker for inducible lincosamide resistance. If the clinician is considering clindamycin, an erythromycin-clindamycin "D-zone" test is prudent. To perform a D-test, clindaymcin and erythromycin disks are placed close together on a culture plate. If inducible lincosamide resistance is present, the zone of inhibition around the clindamycin disk is flattened on the side toward the erythromycin disk. This results in a zone of inhibition resembling a capital letter D instead of an O.

Rates of inducible lincosamide resistance vary widely around the country. Studies in Houston indicate rates of 2% to 8%. In Baltimore, 43% of erythromycin-resistant staphylococci demonstrate inducible lincosamide resistance, and in Chicago, 94% demonstrate inducible lincosamide resistance [41,42,45–47]. Although the rate of inducible resistance is currently relatively low in Houston, surveillance data indicate that the rate of clindamycin resistance is increasing in that location [48]. In contrast, inducible resistance may be becoming less common in Dallas. One study showed inducible resistance among erythromycin-resistant and clindamycin-susceptible CA-MRSA in Dallas dropped from 93% in 1999 to 7% in 2002 [49].

In some areas, CA-MRSA strains have been shown to be less likely than MSSA to demonstrate inducible lincosamide resistance. In Philadelphia,

68% of "clindamycin susceptible" erythromycin resistant methicillin-sensitive isolates were D-test positive in contrast to only 12.3% of the MRSA isolates [50]. In contrast, a study in northern Taiwan, found that 100% of 17 CA-MRSA cases demonstrated the macrolide-lincosamide-streptogramin-constitutive phenotype and the ermB gene [51]. Taken together, the data suggest that clindamycin may not be the best antibiotic choice in many geographic areas.

Many cutaneous abscesses respond to drainage alone, and most of the remaining CA-MRSA infections can be treated with trimethoprim–sulfamethoxazole or a tetracycline, such as doxycycline or minocycline. For serious infections, other antibiotics may play a role. Options include vancomycin, fluoroquinolones, daptomycin, quinupristin–dalfopristin, newer-generation carbapenems, and linezolid.

Fluoroquinolones, such as levofloxacin, moxifloxacin, and gatifloxacin, are effective orally and generally provide adequate coverage for CA-MRSA. Unfortunately, resistance is emerging among both MSSA and MRSA isolates, and data suggest that overuse of flouroquinolones promotes emergence of MRSA strains in the community [52–58]. Linezolid, an oxazolidinone, is useful for severe refractory MRSA infections and can also be administered orally [59]. In some severely ill patients, linezolid therapy has proved to be more effective than vancomycin, but resistance is emerging and the drug should be reserved for serious infections [60–63].

Vancomycin remains an effective drug for many serious infections. Although it must be administered parenterally, skilled home nurses are very adept at administering the drug. Daptomycin has been used effectively in serious MRSA infections, but must be given parenterally [64–66]. Daptomycin resistance has been reported, and disk diffusion testing may fail to predict clinical outcome [67,68]. Most MRSA isolates are susceptible to quinupristin–dalfopristin, another parental agent [69–71]. Unfortunately, some strains have already developed resistance to quinupristin–dalfopristin [72]. Newer carbapenems, such as meropenem, panipenem, and ertapenem, have demonstrated activity against MRSA and synergism with vancomycin [73,74]. Tigecycline, a derivative of minocycline, shows efficacy against MRSA isolates resistant to other tetracyclines [75]. A new cephalosporin, ceftobiprole medocaril, may be comparable in efficacy to vancomycin [76].

Management of skin and nasal colonization

In all patients with MRSA infection, nasal and skin surface colonization should be addressed to prevent recurrent infection. Skin surface colonization can be addressed by topical antiseptics, such as chlorhexidine, povidone iodine, quaternary ammonium compounds, triclosan, and Dakin's solution. Chlorhexidine gluconate is the most widely used topical antiseptic in health care settings. It generally has good activity against staphylococci, although some MRSA isolates are less sensitive than MSSA isolates [77–79]. The resistance shown in some MRSA strains can be overcome by using hand disinfectants containing both alcohol and chlorhexidine [80]. Ethanol has shown efficacy in a study of fomite sterilization. The study compared povidone iodine, benzalkonium chloride, chlorhexidine gluconate, and ethanol. Seventy percent ethanol proved to be the most effective agent, eradicating both MRSA and MSSA in <3 minutes. In this study, chlorhexidine gluconate was the least effective of the four disinfectants [81].

Some MRSA isolates exhibiting low-level resistance to chlorhexidine have shown resistance to the quaternary ammonium compounds [82].

Povidone iodine is another widely used topical biocide in the health care setting. Although published data are limited, some show good activity against both MRSA and MSSA isolates [78].

Alcohol has also been used as an active ingredient, and alcohol-based handrubs containing 62.5% ethyl alcohol have been shown to reduce infection rates when paired with an antimicrobial soap containing 0.3% triclosan. The intervention resulted in a 21% decrease in new nosocomial MRSA infections (90 to 71 isolates per year; $P = .01$) [83].

Triclosan-based products are gaining market share, and have proved helpful in controlling MRSA in health care settings [84–86]. Some triclosan resistance has been documented and, as with chlorhexidine, some MRSA isolates are less sensitive than MSSA isolates [87,88].

Although mupirocin is commonly used to treat staphylococcal nasal carriage, resistant strains have emerged [89]. The efficacy of mupirocin in clearing nasal colonization may be overestimated. In a double-blind, placebo-controlled trial, nasal eradication was only 44% in the mupirocin group compared with 23% in the placebo group [90]. As nasal carriage represents a major reservoir of CA-MRSA colonization, there is an urgent need for additional effective options to treat colonization.

Summary

CA-MRSA strains have emerged as an important group of pathogens. Most infections present as cutaneous abscess and most of these may respond to drainage alone. Sulfonamide and tetracycline antibiotics remain valuable agents for most CA-MRSA infections, but inducible resistance to clindamycin is problematic in some areas. Linezolid, and the newer parenteral antibiotics should be reserved for serious infections.

References

[1] Udo EE, Pearman JW, Grubb WB. Genetic analysis of community isolates of methicillin-resistant *Staphylococcus aureus* in Western Australia. J Hosp Infect 1993;25:97–108.

[2] Lu D, Holtom P. Community-acquired methicillin-resistant Staphylococcus aureus, a new player in sports medicine. Curr Sports Med Rep 2005;4(5): 265–70.

[3] Weber JT. Community-associated methicillin-resistant Staphylococcus aureus. Clin Infect Dis 2005; 41(Suppl 4):S269–72.

[4] Charlebois ED, Perdreau-Remington F, Kreiswirth B, et al. Origins of community strains of methicillin-resistant Staphylococcus aureus. Clin Infect Dis 2004;39(1):47–54.

[5] Mathews WC, Caperna JC, Barber RE, et al. Incidence of and risk factors for clinically significant methicillin-resistant Staphylococcus aureus infection in a cohort of HIV-infected adults. J Acquir Immune Defic Syndr 2005;40(2):155–60.

[6] Naimi TS, LeDell KH, Como-Sabetti K, et al. Comparison of community- and health care-associated methicillin-resistant Staphylococcus aureus infection. JAMA 2003;290(22):2976–84.

[7] Kowalski TJ, Berbari EF, Osmon DR. Epidemiology, treatment, and prevention of community-acquired methicillin-resistant Staphylococcus aureus infections. Mayo Clin Proc 2005;80(9):1201–7.

[8] Iyer S, Jones DH. Community-acquired methicillin-resistant Staphylococcus aureus skin infection: a retrospective analysis of clinical presentation and treatment of a local outbreak. J Am Acad Dermatol 2004;50(6):854–8.

[9] Diep BA, Sensabaugh GF, Somboona NS, et al. Widespread skin and soft-tissue infections due to two methicillin-resistant Staphylococcus aureus strains harboring the genes for Panton-Valentine leucocidin. J Clin Microbiol 2004;42(5): 2080–4.

[10] Cohen PR. Cutaneous community-acquired methicillin-resistant Staphylococcus aureus infection in participants of athletic activities. South Med J 2005; 98(6):596–602.

[11] Frazee BW, Lynn J, Charlebois ED, et al. High prevalence of methicillin-resistant Staphylococcus aureus in emergency department skin and soft tissue infections. Ann Emerg Med 2005;45(3):311–20.

[12] Carleton HA, Diep BA, Charlebois ED, et al. Community-adapted methicillin-resistant Staphylococcus aureus (MRSA): population dynamics of an expanding community reservoir of MRSA. J Infect Dis 2004;190(10):1730–8.

[13] Tirabassi MV, Wadie G, Moriarty KP, et al. Geographic information system localization of community-acquired MRSA soft tissue abscesses. J Pediatr Surg 2005;40(6):962–5.

[14] Purcell K, Fergie J. Epidemic of community-acquired methicillin-resistant Staphylococcus aureus infections: a 14-year study at Driscoll Children's Hospital. Arch Pediatr Adolesc Med 2005;159(10): 980–5.

[15] Said-Salim B, Mathema B, Kreiswirth BN. Community-acquired methicillin-resistant Staphylococcus aureus: an emerging pathogen. Infect Control Hosp Epidemiol 2003;24(6):451–5.

[16] Stemper ME, Shukla SK, Reed KD. Emergence and spread of community-associated methicillin-resistant Staphylococcus aureus in rural Wisconsin, 1989 to 1999. J Clin Microbiol 2004;42(12): 5673–80.

[17] Baggett HC, Hennessy TW, Leman R, et al. An outbreak of community-onset methicillin-resistant Staphylococcus aureus skin infections in southwestern Alaska. Infect Control Hosp Epidemiol 2003; 24(6):397–402.

[18] Dietrich DW, Auld DB, Mermel LA. Community-acquired methicillin-resistant Staphylococcus aureus in southern New England children. Pediatrics 2004;113(4):e347–52.

[19] Kourbatova EV, Halvosa JS, King MD, et al. Emergence of community-associated methicillin-resistant Staphylococcus aureus USA 300 clone as a cause of health care-associated infections among patients with prosthetic joint infections. Am J Infect Control 2005;33(7):385–91.

[20] Naas T, Fortineau N, Spicq C, et al. Three-year survey of community-acquired methicillin-resistant Staphylococcus aureus producing Panton-Valentine leukocidin in a French university hospital. J Hosp Infect 2005;61:321–9.

[21] Saiman L, O'Keefe M, Graham PL 3rd, et al. Hospital transmission of community-acquired methicillin-resistant Staphylococcus aureus among postpartum women. Clin Infect Dis 2003;37(10):1313–9.

[22] Eckhardt C, Halvosa JS, Ray SM, et al. Transmission of methicillin-resistant Staphylococcus aureus in the neonatal intensive care unit from a patient with community-acquired disease. Infect Control Hosp Epidemiol 2003;24(6):460–1.

[23] Salgado CD, Farr BM, Calfee DP. Community-acquired methicillin-resistant Staphylococcus aureus:

a meta-analysis of prevalence and risk factors. Clin Infect Dis 2003;36(2):131–9.

[24] Lesens O, Hansmann Y, Brannigan E, et al. Health-care-associated Staphylococcus aureus bacteremia and the risk for methicillin resistance: is the Centers for Disease Control and Prevention definition for community-acquired bacteremia still appropriate? Infect Control Hosp Epidemiol 2005;26(2):204–9.

[25] Baggett HC, Hennessy TW, Rudolph K, et al. Community-onset methicillin-resistant Staphylococcus aureus associated with antibiotic use and the cytotoxin Panton-Valentine leukocidin during a furunculosis outbreak in rural Alaska. J Infect Dis 2004; 189(9):1565–73.

[26] Calfee DP, Durbin LJ, Germanson TP, et al. Spread of methicillin-resistant Staphylococcus aureus (MRSA) among household contacts of individuals with nosocomially acquired MRSA. Infect Control Hosp Epidemiol 2003;24(6):422–6.

[27] Ellis MW, Hospenthal DR, Dooley DP, et al. Natural history of community-acquired methicillin-resistant Staphylococcus aureus colonization and infection in soldiers. Clin Infect Dis 2004;39(7): 971–9.

[28] Laibl VR, Sheffield JS, Roberts S, et al. Clinical presentation of community-acquired methicillin-resistant Staphylococcus aureus in pregnancy. Obstet Gynecol 2005;106(3):461–5.

[29] Miller LG, Perdreau-Remington F, Rieg G, et al. Necrotizing fasciitis caused by community-associated methicillin-resistant Staphylococcus aureus in Los Angeles. N Engl J Med 2005;352(14):1445–53.

[30] Gonzalez BE, Hulten KG, Dishop MK, et al. Pulmonary manifestations in children with invasive community-acquired Staphylococcus aureus infection. Clin Infect Dis 2005;41(5):583–90.

[31] Gonzalez BE, Martinez-Aguilar G, Hulten KG, et al. Severe Staphylococcal sepsis in adolescents in the era of community-acquired methicillin-resistant Staphylococcus aureus. Pediatrics 2005;115(3): 642–8.

[32] Fridkin SK, Hageman JC, Morrison M, et al. Active Bacterial Core Surveillance Program of the Emerging Infections Program Network. Methicillin-resistant Staphylococcus aureus disease in three communities. N Engl J Med 2005;352(14): 1436–44.

[33] Young DM, Harris HW, Charlebois ED, et al. An epidemic of methicillin-resistant Staphylococcus aureus soft tissue infections among medically underserved patients. Arch Surg 2004;139(9):947–51.

[34] Lee MC, Rios AM, Aten MF, et al. Management and outcome of children with skin and soft tissue abscesses caused by community-acquired methicillin-resistant Staphylococcus aureus. Pediatr Infect Dis J 2004;23(2):123–7.

[35] Rutar T, Zwick OM, Cockerham KP, et al. Bilateral blindness from orbital cellulitis caused by community-acquired methicillin-resistant Staphylococcus aureus. Am J Ophthalmol 2005;140(4):740–2.

[36] Segreti J. Efficacy of current agents used in the treatment of gram-positive infections and the consequences of resistance. Clin Microbiol Infect 2005; (Suppl 3):29–35.

[37] Takizawa Y, Taneike I, Nakagawa S, et al. A Panton-Valentine leucocidin (PVL)-positive community-acquired methicillin-resistant Staphylococcus aureus (MRSA) strain, another such strain carrying a multiple-drug resistance plasmid, and other more-typical PVL-negative MRSA strains found in Japan. J Clin Microbiol 2005;43(7):3356–63.

[38] Boyle-Vavra S, Ereshefsky B, Wang CC, et al. Successful multiresistant community-associated methicillin-resistant Staphylococcus aureus lineage from Taipei, Taiwan, that carries either the novel Staphylococcal chromosome cassette mec (SCCmec) type VT or SCCmec type IV. J Clin Microbiol 2005; 43(9):4719–30.

[39] Chen CJ, Huang YC, Chiu CH, et al. Clinical features and genotyping analysis of community-acquired methicillin-resistant Staphylococcus aureus infections in Taiwanese children. Pediatr Infect Dis J 2005;24(1):40–5.

[40] Braun L, Craft D, Williams R, et al. Increasing clindamycin resistance among methicillin-resistant Staphylococcus aureus in 57 northeast United States military treatment facilities. Pediatr Infect Dis J 2005;24(7):622–6.

[41] Martinez-Aguilar G, Hammerman WA, Mason EO Jr, et al. Clindamycin treatment of invasive infections caused by community-acquired, methicillin-resistant and methicillin-susceptible Staphylococcus aureus in children. Pediatr Infect Dis J 2003;22(7): 593–8.

[42] Lewis JS 2nd, Jorgensen JH. Inducible clindamycin resistance in Staphylococci: should clinicians and microbiologists be concerned? Clin Infect Dis 2005; 40(2):280–5.

[43] Buescher ES. Community-acquired methicillin-resistant Staphylococcus aureus in pediatrics. Curr Opin Pediatr 2005;17(1):67–70.

[44] Marcinak JF, Frank AL. Treatment of community-acquired methicillin-resistant Staphylococcus aureus in children. Curr Opin Infect Dis 2003;16(3):265–9.

[45] Frank AL, Marcinak JF, Mangat PD, et al. Clindamycin treatment of methicillin-resistant Staphylococcus aureus infections in children. Pediatr Infect Dis J 2002;21:530–4.

[46] Siberry GK, Tekle T, Carroll K, et al. Failure of clindamycin treatment of methicillin-resistant Staphylococcus aureus expressing inducible clindamycin resistance in vitro. Clin Infect Dis 2003;37:1257–60.

[47] Sattler CA, Mason EO Jr, Kaplan SL. Prospective comparison of risk factors and demographic and clinical characteristics of community-acquired, methicillin-resistant versus methicillin-susceptible

Staphylococcus aureus infection in children. Pediatr Infect Dis J 2002;21:910–7.

[48] Kaplan SL, Hulten KG, Gonzalez BE, et al. Three-year surveillance of community-acquired Staphylococcus aureus infections in children. Clin Infect Dis 2005;40(12):1785–91.

[49] Chavez-Bueno S, Bozdogan B, Katz K, et al. Inducible clindamycin resistance and molecular epidemiologic trends of pediatric community-acquired methicillin-resistant Staphylococcus aureus in Dallas, Texas. Antimicrob Agents Chemother 2005; 49(6):2283–8.

[50] Levin TP, Suh B, Axelrod P, et al. Potential clindamycin resistance in clindamycin-susceptible, erythromycin-resistant Staphylococcus aureus: report of a clinical failure. Antimicrob Agents Chemother 2005;49:1222–4.

[51] Wang CC, Lo WT, Chu ML, et al. Epidemiological typing of community-acquired methicillin-resistant Staphylococcus aureus isolates from children in Taiwan. Clin Infect Dis 2004;39(4):481–7.

[52] Marangon FB, Miller D, Muallem MS, et al. Ciprofloxacin and levofloxacin resistance among methicillin-sensitive Staphylococcus aureus isolates from keratitis and conjunctivitis. Am J Ophthalmol 2004;137(3):453–8.

[53] Horii T, Suzuki Y, Monji A, et al. Detection of mutations in quinolone resistance-determining regions in levofloxacin- and methicillin-resistant Staphylococcus aureus: effects of the mutations on fluoroquinolone MICs. Diagn Microbiol Infect Dis 2003; 46(2):139–45.

[54] Venezia RA, Domaracki BE, Evans AM, et al. Selection of high-level oxacillin resistance in heteroresistant Staphylococcus aureus by fluoroquinolone exposure. J Antimicrob Chemother 2001;48(3):375–81.

[55] Harbarth S, Liassine N, Dharan S, et al. Risk factors for persistent carriage of methicillin-resistant Staphylococcus aureus. Clin Infect Dis 2000;31(6):1380–5.

[56] Weber SG, Gold HS, Hooper DC, et al. Fluoroquinolones and the risk for methicillin-resistant Staphylococcus aureus in hospitalized patients. Emerg Infect Dis 2003;9(11):1415–22.

[57] MacDougall C, Harpe SE, Powell JP, et al. Pseudomonas aeruginosa, Staphylococcus aureus, and fluoroquinolone use. Emerg Infect Dis 2005;11(8): 1197–204.

[58] MacDougall C, Powell JP, Johnson CK, et al. Hospital and community fluoroquinolone use and resistance in Staphylococcus aureus and Escherichia coli in 17 US hospitals. Clin Infect Dis 2005;41(4):435–40.

[59] Wilson SE. Clinical trial results with linezolid, an oxazolidinone, in the treatment of soft tissue and postoperative gram-positive infections. Surg Infect (Larchmt) 2001;2(1):25–35.

[60] Machado AR, Arns Cda C, Follador W, et al. Cost-effectiveness of linezolid versus vancomycin in mechanical ventilation-associated nosocomial pneumonia caused by methicillin-resistant Staphylococcus aureus. Braz J Infect Dis 2005;9(3):191–200.

[61] Weigelt J, Itani K, Stevens D, et al. Linezolid CSSTI Study Group. Linezolid versus vancomycin in treatment of complicated skin and soft tissue infections. Antimicrob Agents Chemother 2005;49(6):2260–6.

[62] Sharpe JN, Shively EH, Polk HC Jr. Clinical and economic outcomes of oral linezolid versus intravenous vancomycin in the treatment of MRSA-complicated, lower-extremity skin and soft-tissue infections caused by methicillin-resistant Staphylococcus aureus. Am J Surg 2005;189(4):425–8.

[63] Li JZ, Willke RJ, Rittenhouse BE, et al. Effect of linezolid versus vancomycin on length of hospital stay in patients with complicated skin and soft tissue infections caused by known or suspected methicillin-resistant staphylococci: results from a randomized clinical trial. Surg Infect (Larchmt) 2003;4(1):57–70.

[64] Tally FP, Zeckel M, Wasilewski MM, et al. Daptomycin: a novel agent for gram-positive infections. Expert Opin Investig Drugs 1999;8(8):1223–38.

[65] Hsueh PR, Chen WH, Teng LJ, et al. Nosocomial infections due to methicillin-resistant Staphylococcus aureus and vancomycin-resistant enterococci at a university hospital in Taiwan from 1991 to 2003: resistance trends, antibiotic usage and in vitro activities of newer antimicrobial agents. Int J Antimicrob Agents 2005;26(1):43–9.

[66] LaPlante KL, Rybak MJ. Daptomycin—a novel antibiotic against gram-positive pathogens. Expert Opin Pharmacother 2004;5(11):2321–31.

[67] Mangili A, Bica I, Snydman DR, et al. Daptomycin-resistant, methicillin-resistant Staphylococcus aureus bacteremia. Clin Infect Dis 2005;40(7): 1058–60.

[68] Hayden MK, Rezai K, Hayes RA, et al. Development of Daptomycin resistance in vivo in methicillin-resistant Staphylococcus aureus. J Clin Microbiol 2005;43(10):5285–7.

[69] Sander A, Beiderlinden M, Schmid EN, et al. Clinical experience with quinupristin-dalfopristin as rescue treatment of critically ill patients infected with methicillin-resistant staphylococci. Intensive Care Med 2002;28(8):1157–60.

[70] Goff DA, Sierawski SJ. Clinical experience of quinupristin-dalfopristin for the treatment of antimicrobial-resistant gram-positive infections. Pharmacotherapy 2002;22(6):748–58.

[71] Brown J, Freeman BB 3rd. Combining quinupristin/dalfopristin with other agents for resistant infections. Ann Pharmacother 2004;38(4):677–85.

[72] Luh KT, Hsueh PR, Teng LJ, et al. Quinupristin-dalfopristin resistance among gram-positive bacteria in Taiwan. Antimicrob Agents Chemother. 2000 Dec;44(12):3374–3380.

[73] Imamura H, Ohtake N, Jona H, et al. Dicationic dithiocarbamate carbapenems with anti-MRSA activity. Bioorg Med Chem 2001;9(6):1571–8.

[74] Kobayashi Y. Study of the synergism between carbapenems and vancomycin or teicoplanin against MRSA, focusing on S-4661, a carbapenem newly developed in Japan. J Infect Chemother 2005;11(5):259–61.

[75] Petersen PJ, Jacobus NV, Weiss WJ, et al. In vitro and in vivo antibacterial activities of a novel glycylcycline, the 9-t-butylglycylamido derivative of minocycline (GAR-936). Antimicrob Agents Chemother 1999;43(4):738–44.

[76] Vaudaux P, Gjinovci A, Bento M, et al. Intensive therapy with ceftobiprole medocaril of experimental foreign-body infection by methicillin-resistant Staphylococcus aureus. Antimicrob Agents Chemother 2005;49(9):3789–93.

[77] Kanazawa K, Ueda Y. Bactericial activity of chlorhexidine gluconate against recent clinical isolates of various bacterial species in Japan. Jpn J Antibiot 2004;57(5):449–64.

[78] Block C, Robenshtok E, Simhon A, et al. Evaluation of chlorhexidine and povidone iodine activity against methicillin-resistant Staphylococcus aureus and vancomycin-resistant Enterococcus faecalis using a surface test. J Hosp Infect 2000;46(2):147–52.

[79] Zhang YH, Liu XY, Zhu LL, et al. Study on the resistance of methicillin-resistant staphylococcus aureus to iodophor and chlorhexidine. Zhonghua Liu Xing Bing Xue Za Zhi 2004;25(3):248–50 [in Chinese].

[80] Kampf G, Jarosch R, Ruden H. Limited effectiveness of chlorhexidine based hand disinfectants against methicillin-resistant Staphylococcus aureus (MRSA). J Hosp Infect 1998;38(4):297–303.

[81] Suzuki J, Komatsuzawa H, Kozai K, et al. In vitro susceptibility of Staphylococcus aureus including MRSA to four disinfectants. ASDC J Dent Child 1997;64(4):260–3.

[82] Suller MT, Russell AD. Antibiotic and biocide resistance in methicillin-resistant Staphylococcus aureus and vancomycin-resistant enterococcus. J Hosp Infect 1999;43(4):281–91.

[83] Gordin FM, Schultz ME, Huber RA, et al. Reduction in nosocomial transmission of drug-resistant bacteria after introduction of an alcohol-based handrub. Infect Control Hosp Epidemiol 2005;26(7):650–3.

[84] Zafar AB, Butler RC, Reese DJ, et al. Use of 0.3% triclosan (Bacti-Stat) to eradicate an outbreak of methicillin-resistant Staphylococcus aureus in a neonatal nursery. Am J Infect Control 1995;23(3):200–8.

[85] Webster J, Faoagali JL, Cartwright D. Elimination of methicillin-resistant Staphylococcus aureus from a neonatal intensive care unit after hand washing with triclosan. J Paediatr Child Health 1994;30(1):59–64.

[86] Webster J. Handwashing in a neonatal intensive care nursery: product acceptability and effectiveness of chlorhexidine gluconate 4% and triclosan 1%. J Hosp Infect 1992;21(2):137–41.

[87] Brenwald NP, Fraise AP. Triclosan resistance in methicillin-resistant Staphylococcus aureus (MRSA). J Hosp Infect 2003;55(2):141–4.

[88] Bamber AI, Neal TJ. An assessment of triclosan susceptibility in methicillin-resistant and methicillin-sensitive Staphylococcus aureus. J Hosp Infect 1999;41(2):107–9.

[89] Mulvey MR, MacDougall L, Cholin B, et al. Saskatchewan CA-MRSA Study Group. Community-associated methicillin-resistant Staphylococcus aureus, Canada. Emerg Infect Dis 2005;11(6):844–50.

[90] Harbarth S, Dharan S, Liassine N, et al. Randomized, placebo-controlled, double-blind trial to evaluate the efficacy of mupirocin for eradicating carriage of methicillin-resistant Staphylococcus aureus. Antimicrob Agents Chemother 1999;43(6):1412–6.

Dermatol Clin 25 (2007) 165–183

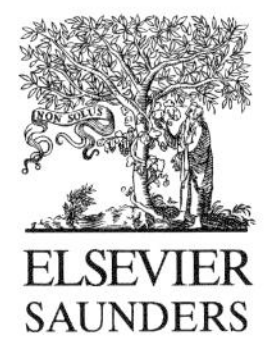

DERMATOLOGIC
CLINICS

Advances in Topical and Systemic Antifungals

Alexandra Y. Zhang, MD[a], William L. Camp, MD, MPH[b],
Boni E. Elewski, MD[a],*

[a]Department of Dermatology, University of Alabama at Birmingham, EFH 414, 1530 3rd Avenue South,
Birmingham, AL 35294, USA
[b]Department of Medicine, University of Alabama at Birmingham, 1530 3rd Avenue South,
Birmingham, AL 35294, USA

Superficial fungal infections of the hair, skin, and nails are common yet often difficult to treat. Dermatophytes are one of the most common causes of tinea (capitis, manuum, pedis, cruris, corporis, barbae) and onychomycosis. Candidal infections and pityriasis versicolor, caused by *Malassezia furfur*, a lipophilic yeast, are also among the most widespread superficial cutaneous fungal infections. Topical antifungal agents are compounded into different types of vehicles, such as creams, lotions, gels, or sprays. When applied to the skin surface, they readily penetrate into the stratum corneum to either kill the fungi or inhibit their growth, achieving clinical and mycologic eradication. The main classes of topical antifungal treatment modalities include the polyenes, the azoles, and the allylamine/benzylamines (Table 1). Other topical antifungal agents include ciclopirox, a hydroxypyridone, thiocarbonate, haloprogin, and selenium sulfide.

Oral or systemic antifungals are often used for the treatment of onychomycosis, superficial and systemic candidiasis, and prophylaxis and treatment of invasive fungal infections. Amphotericin B, flucytosine, itraconazole, and ketoconazole have been the mainstream systemic antifungal therapies for many years; however, drug toxicity, the emergence of resistant strains, and low efficacy have limited their use clinically. During the past two decades, various new antifungal agents with improved absorption and efficacy have demonstrated significant therapeutic potential. Voriconazole, micafungin, caspofungin, and lipid formulations of amphotericin B have arrived on the market and have broadened clinicians' choices in the treatment of systemic invasive fungal infections.

Polyenes

The polyene antifungal agents were first developed in the late 1950s. They are produced by fermentation by *Streptomyces* species. Structurally, polyene antifungal agents are characterized by a macrolide ring of carbon atoms with conjugated double bonds. In general, polyene antifungals have higher affinity to ergosterol, a fungal cell membrane sterol, than they do to human cell cholesterol. They bind irreversibly to ergosterol, resulting in a change of membrane permeability and subsequent leakage of intracellular components by creating pores in the cell membrane, destroying the fungal cell [1].

Amphotericin B and nystatin are the two mainstream polyene antifungal agents that are widely used clinically in the treatment of superficial and systemic fungal infections. They are ineffective against infections caused by dermatophytes.

Nystatin

History

In 1950, Hazen and Brown [2] developed the antifungal agent nystatin through a long-distance collaboration. Named after the New York State Department of Health, nystatin first became available in practical form as a specific antifungal antibiotic in 1954 following US Food and Drug Administration (FDA) approval.

---

* Corresponding author.
E-mail address: beelewski@aol.com (B.E. Elewski).

Table 1
Classification and mechanism of action of antifungal antibiotics

Class	Representative drugs	Mechanism of action	Antifungal effects
Polyenes	Nystatin	Interaction with ergosterol, formation of aqueous channels, increased membrane permeability and subsequent leakage of intracellular	Fungistatic and Fungicidal
	Amphotericin B	components	Fungicidal
Azoles		Inhibition of fungal lanosterol 14-α demethylase resulting in depletion of ergosterol and accumulation of toxic sterols in the fungal cell membrane	Fungistatic
Imidazoles	Clotrimazole		
	Econazole		
	Ketoconazole		
	Miconazole		
	Oxiconazole		
Trizoles	Fluconazole		
	Itraconazole		
	Voriconazole		*Candida:* time-dependent fungistatic *Aspergillus:* time-dependent slow fungicidal
Allylamines	Naftine	Interferes with synthesis of ergosterol by inhibiting squalene 2,3-epoxidase that is responsible to convert squalene to squalene oxide	Dermatophytes: fungicidal *Candida:* fungistatic
	Terbinafine		
Benzylamines	Butenafine		
Echinocandins	Caspofungin	Blocks 1,3-β-D-glucan synthase resulting in depletion of cell wall glucan and osmotic instability	Candida: fungicidal Aspigillus: fungistatic
	Micafungin		
Hydroxypyridone	Ciclopirox	Inhibition of essential enzymes by creating a large polyvalent cation through chelation, thus interfering with mitochondrial electron transport processes and energy production.	Fungicidal and fungistatic
Other antifungals	Griseofulvin	Inhibition of fungal cell mitosis and nucleic acid synthesis and interference with the function of spindles and cytoplasmic microtubules by binding to alpha and beta tubulin	Fungistatic

Mechanism of action

Nystatin is a polyene derivative produced by *Streptomyces albidus* and *S noursei* that acts by irreversibly binding to ergosterol in the fungal cell membrane, creating a pore in the membrane with a resultant leakage of essential intracellular components that kills the fungal cell [2,3].

Absorption

Nystatin is limited to topical use owing to its severe toxicity when administered intravenously. It is ineffective orally. Absorption of nystatin from intact skin, mucous membranes, and the gastrointestinal tract is insignificant [4].

Pregnancy category

Nystatin for topical indications is rated pregnancy category B, and oral nystatin is in pregnancy category C.

Available forms

Nystatin is available as a cream, ointment, and powder for twice daily cutaneous application. It is also available as a liquid, suspension, and pastille used four to five times a day for the treatment of oral candidiasis.

Clinical indication

Nystatin is both fungistatic and fungicidal in vitro. Clinically, topical nystatin has demonstrated broad antifungal activity in treating mucocutaneous fungal infections caused by *Candida* species such as *C albicans, C parapsilosis, C krusei,* and *C tropicalis* [5]. Nystatin is not indicated for the treatment of dermatomycosis caused by dermatophytes.

Adverse effects

Nystatin is well tolerated by most patients. The most common adverse effect includes allergic contact dermatitis [6]. Hypersensitivity reactions including Stevens-Johnson syndrome have been reported rarely [7]. Large oral doses have occasionally caused gastrointestinal distress such as nausea, vomiting, and diarrhea [8].

Amphotericin B

History

Discovered in 1956 by Gold and colleagues [9], amphotericin B was obtained from a filamentous bacterium, *Streptomyces nodosus.* The drug is currently available in several formulations including plain amphotericin B deoxycholate, amphotericin B colloidal dispersion, a cholesteryl sulfate complex, a lipid complex, and a liposomal formulation [10]. The lipid formulations have been developed to decrease the toxicity and improve tolerability for patients.

Mechanism of action

As is true for other polyene antifungals, amphotericin B binds to ergosterol of susceptible fungi, forming a pore that leads to intracellular component leakage and subsequent fungal cell death.

Absorption

Gastrointestinal absorption of amphotericin B is insignificant. Its bioavailability achieves 100% by intravenous infusion.

Pregnancy category

Amphotericin B is rated pregnancy category B.

Available forms

Amphotericin B is available as an intravenous infusion.

Clinical indication

Amphotericin B exhibits broad-spectrum antifungal activity against many species of fungi in vitro, including *Blastomyces dermatitidis, Cryptococcus neoformans, Coccidioides immitis, Candida* spp, *Histoplasma capsulatum, Rhodotorula* spp, *Sporothrix schenckii, Mucor mucedo,* and *Aspergillus fumigatus.* Some species, such as *Pseudallescheria boydii* and *Fusarium, Trichosporon, Geotrichum,* and *Scedosporium,* are often resistant or not susceptible to amphotericin B [11]. Clinically, amphotericin B has been used for the treatment of invasive fungal infections.

Adverse effects

An acute hypersensitivity reaction may occur 1 to 3 hours after infusion that may partially contribute to an increased synthesis of prostaglandin and histamine liberation that results in fever, chills, nausea, vomiting, headache, hypotension, dyspnea, and tachypnea. Starting with a low initial dose may help to decrease the occurrence and severity of the reaction. Nephrotoxicity is a major adverse effect and can be irreversible. Hepatotoxicity, electrolyte imbalances, leukopenia, thrombocytopenia, cardiac arrhythmias and cardiac failure, and cutaneous drug eruptions may also occur [12]. When amphotericin B is delivered in lipid formulations, the adverse effects are generally diminished [12,13].

Azoles

Azole antifungals are composed of the imidazoles and triazoles. Triazoles differ from imidazoles by having three instead of two nitrogen atoms in the azole ring. Azoles work through a common mechanism of action. They are fungistatic but not fungicidal, except at very high concentrations. Azoles selectively inhibit the synthesis of ergosterol, an essential component of fungal cell membrane, by interacting with fungal lanosterol 14-α demethylase, a cytochrome P-450 dependent enzyme that converts lanosterol to ergosterol. Depletion of ergosterol and accumulation of 14-α-methylated sterols interferes with the function of ergosterol, causes increased permeability and rigidity of fungal cell membrane, and disrupts the enzymes bound to fungal cell membrane, inhibiting fungal growth and replication. Unlike the process in fungal cells, human cell demethylation is much less sensitive to the inhibition of azoles [1]. Fluconazole, itraconazole, ketoconazole, voriconazole, posaconazole, and ravuconazole are used for systemic treatment.

Clotrimazole

History

The first topical antifungal imidazole, clotrimazole, was developed in the late 1960s by Plempel [14], who was a chief mycologist of the Bayer AG (Germany).

Mechanism

Clotrimazole is an imidazole derivative that demonstrates a broad spectrum of antimycotic activity. Like other azoles, it operates by inhibiting 14-α demethylase, interrupting the synthesis of fungal ergosterol that results in increased permeability of the cell membrane. In addition, clotrimazole may impair membrane phospholipid synthesis, accelerate important intracellular ion efflux, cause a breakdown of cellular nucleic acids, and inhibit endogenous respiration. The end result is cessation of cell division and growth [1].

Absorption

Clotrimazole is absorbed poorly when administered orally. Absorption into intact skin after topical application is extremely low. The concentration of clotrimazole measured is 100 $\mu g/cm^3$ in the stratum corneum, 0.5 to 1 $\mu g/cm^3$ in the dermis, and 0.1 $\mu g/cm^3$ in the subcutaneous fat, respectively, after application of 1% clotrimazole cream and solution to intact and inflamed skin (data on file, Schering Corp., Kenilworth, New Jersey, 1993).

Available forms

Clotrimazole is available as a cream or ointment for the treatment of cutaneous fungal infections. It is also available as a spray, powder, liquid, solution, suppository, and lozenge for the treatment of oral and vaginal candidiasis.

Pregnancy category

Topical clotrimazole is rated pregnancy category B.

Clinical indication

Clotrimazole is active against most *Trichophyton*, *Epidermophyton*, and *Microsporum* species [15]. Clinically, twice daily application of clotrimazole has been used in the topical treatment of tinea corporis, tinea pedis, tinea versicolor, and oral and mucocutaneous candidiasis [16,17].

Adverse effects

In general, clotrimazole is well tolerated by most patients. Occasionally, patients may experience irritation with a burning sensation at the site of application. Allergic contact dermatitis with erythema, edema, urticaria, and pruritus has been reported rarely (data on file, Schering Corp., Kenilworth, New Jersey, 1993).

Econazole

History

Econazole, a derivative of imidazole, was first synthesized by Janssen Pharmaceutica in 1969 [18].

Mechanism

Like other azoles, econazole inhibits 14-α demethylase and interrupts conversion of lanosterol to ergosterol, causing cessation of fungal cell growth [1].

Absorption

Systemic absorption of econazole is extremely low after topical application to the skin. Although most econazole remains on the skin surface after application, concentrations of econazole that have been found in the stratum corneum exceed the minimum inhibitory concentration for dermatophytes, and inhibitory concentrations are achieved in the middermis [19].

Clinical indications

Topical application of econazole 1% cream has been used in the treatment of tinea pedis, tinea cruris, and tinea corporis caused by *Trichophyton rubrum*, *T mentagrophytes*, *T tonsurans*, *Microsporum canis*, *M audouini*, *M gypseum*, and *Epidermophyton floccosum*. It is also used in treating cutaneous candidiasis caused by *Candida albicans* and tinea versicolor caused by *Malassezia furfur* [19].

Available forms

Econazole is available as a cream and suppository.

Pregnancy category

Econazole is rated pregnancy category C.

Adverse effects

Most patients tolerate topical econazole well. Only 3% of patients have reported erythema, burning, itching, or stinging during clinical trials. One case of pruritic skin eruption has been reported in literature [20].

Fluconazole

History

Fluconazole, a member of the triazole antifungal family, was approved by the FDA in the early 1990s.

Mechanism

Like other azoles, fluconazole operates by selectively interacting with fungal cell cytochrome P-450 enzyme 14-α demethylase. It inhibits the conversion of lanosterol to ergosterol, causing cessation of fungal cell division and growth [1].

Absorption

Fluconazole is highly water soluble and well absorbed after oral administration. Unlike itraconazole, fluconazole is not influenced by gastric pH. The bioavailability of orally administered fluconazole is over 90% when compared with intravenous administration. Fluconazole predominantly undergoes renal clearance. The dose needs to be adjusted based on creatinine clearance [21].

Clinical indications

Fluconazole exhibits in vitro fungistatic activity against *Candida* species and *Cryptococcus neoformans*. It has also been demonstrated to be active against fungal infections caused by *Aspergillus flavus, A fumigatus, Blastomyces dermatitidis, Coccidioides immitis*, and *Histoplasma capsulatum* in animal models. Clinically, it is indicated in the treatment of vaginal, oropharyngeal, and esophageal candidiasis, candidemia, disseminated candidiasis, and cryptococcal meningitis. Fluconazole is not officially approved for the treatment of onychomycosis in the United States. In off-label use, fluconazole has been found to be effective in the treatment of onychomycosis, tinea corporis, tinea cruris, tinea pedis, tinea capitis, pityriasis versicolor, and cutaneous and chronic mucocutaneous candidiasis [22].

Available forms

Fluconazole is available as a capsule, liquid, powder for solution, and tablets.

Pregnancy category

Fluconazole is rated pregnancy category C.

Adverse effects

The most common adverse effects of fluconazole are mild to moderate in severity, including headache, nausea, abdominal pain, diarrhea, dyspepsia, dizziness, and taste perversion [22]. Several cases of fluconazole induced Q-T prolongation with or without torsade de pointes have been reported in the literature as cardiotoxic effects [23]. In rare cases, anaphylactic reactions including angioedema, Stevens-Johnson syndrome, and toxic epidermal necrolysis have been reported after administration of fluconazole [24].

Interactions

Fluconazole is a potent inhibitor of cytochrome P-450 enzyme activity. It interacts with many drugs whose clearance is dominated by P-450 2C9 or 3A4. As listed in Table 2, coadministration of fluconazole and these drugs may result in elevated plasma concentrations of the drugs that could potentially increase therapeutic effects and side effects; therefore, precautions need to be taken, and appropriate dosage adjustments may be necessary [25].

Itraconazole

History

Itraconazole, a synthetic triazole antifungal agent developed in the late 1980s, has broad-spectrum antifungal activity against various species of dermatophytes, yeast, and dimorphic and filamentous fungi.

Mechanism

Like other azoles, itraconazole selectively inhibits fungal cell cytochrome P-450 enzyme 14-α demethylase, inhibiting the conversion of lanosterol to ergosterol and causing cessation of fungal cell division and growth by interrupting fungal wall synthesis [1].

Absorption

The absolute oral bioavailability of itraconazole is 55%. Absorption of itraconazole can be enhanced by increased gastric pH when taken with a full meal. Itraconazole is highly lipophilic and is metabolized in the liver predominately by the cytochrome P-450 3A4 isoenzyme system (CYP3A4). The metabolites of itraconazole are excreted in the urine and bile [26].

Clinical indications

Like other azole antifungal agents, itraconazole is mainly fungistatic. It demonstrates good in vitro activity against *Candida albicans, Cryptococcus neoformans, Blastomyces dermatitidis, Histoplasma capsulatum, H duboisii, Aspergillus flavus*, and *A fumigatus*. It also has variable activity against *Sporothrix schenckii, Trichophyton* species, *Candida krusei*, and other *Candida* species in vitro. Clinically, it has been approved by the FDA for the treatment of invasive fungal infections in

Table 2
Drugs that have potentially clinically significant pharmacokinetic interactions with systemic itraconazole, ketoconazole, and possibly higher doses of fluconazole (≥ 200 mg/day)

Interaction significance	Potential effects
Life-threatening, concomitant use is contraindicated	
Astemizole	May induce torsade de pointes
Terfenadine	May induce torsade de pointes
Cisapride	Prolongs QT interval that may result in torsade de pointes
Major interactions, concomitant use is contraindicated	
Midazolam	Prolonged sedation
Triazolam	
Lovastatin	Myopathy, rhabdomyolysis
Simvastatin	
Atorvastatin	
Major interactions, concomitant use best avoided or use with caution	
Rifampin	Antifungal inefficacy
Rifabutin	Antifungal inefficacy
Protease inhibitors	Increased effects (voriconazole has no effects on indinavir)
Mild or moderate interaction, precaution to be taken or avoid when used concomitantly	
Digoxin[a]	Digoxin toxicity
Cyclosporin	Increased nephrotoxicity and neurotoxicity
Methylprednisolone	Increased methylprednisolone effects
Warfarin	Enhanced anticoagulant effect
Phenytoin	Increased phenytoin levels or antifungal inefficacy
Oral hypoglycemics[b]	Hypoglycemia
Quinidine	Ototoxicity
Tacrolimus	Increased tacrolimus serum levels
Calcium channel blockers	Edema formation with dihydropyridine type
Carbamazapine	Antifungal inefficacy
H$_2$ blocker antistamines	Inefficacy of itraconazole (capsules) and ketoconazole (tablets)
Isoniazid	Antifungal inefficacy
Proton pump inhibitors	Inefficacy of itraconazole (capsules) and ketoconazole (tablets)

This is not a complete list, please refer to the manufacturer's individual package insert for current information.
[a] Risk of interaction uncertain with fluconazole.
[b] Risk of interaction varies with specific oral hypoglycemic agent and individual azole antifungal agent.

immunocompromised and immunocompetent patients with pulmonary and extrapulmonary blastomycosis, histoplasmosis, and aspergillosis. It is also indicated in the treatment of onychomycosis of the toenails caused by dermatophytes with or without fingernail involvement, or in the treatment of onychomycosis of the fingernails in immunocompetent patients [27]. As an off-label use, itraconazole is also used in the treatment of tinea capitis, corporis, pedis, manuum, and cruris, tinea versicolor, onychomycosis owing to *Candida* spp and nondermatophyte molds, and onychomycosis in children. For the treatment of onychomycosis, a continuous itraconazole regimen (200 mg/day for 6 weeks for fingernails and 12 weeks for toenails) or a pulse regimen (200 mg twice daily for 1 week per month as a single pulse, with two pulses for fingernails and three pulses for toenails) has been used [28–30].

Available forms

Itraconazole is available in capsules and a liquid solution.

Pregnancy category

Itraconazole is rated pregnancy category C.

Adverse effects

The most common adverse effects include gastrointestinal disorders such as dyspepsia, abdominal pain, nausea, and diarrhea, with occasional occurrence of gastritis and hepatitis. Cutaneous side effects include an eruption that tends to occur more often in immunocompromised patients receiving immunosuppressants. Pruritus, urticaria, and Stevens-Johnson syndrome have been rarely reported. Other adverse effects include edema, fatigue, fever, headache, dizziness, hypertension, hypertriglyceridemia, hypokalemia, and, rarely, neutropenia. Of note, itraconazole has been associated with rare cases of liver failure. Monitoring of liver enzymes is recommended when itraconazole is used as a continuous regimen for over 1 month. Itraconazole is contraindicated for the treatment of onychomycosis in patients with congestive heart failure or a history of congestive heart failure [27].

Interactions

Both itraconazole and its bioactive metabolite, hydroxyitraconazole, are potent inhibitors of the CYP3A4 isoenzyme system. The plasma concentration of the drugs primarily metabolized by CYP3A4 (eg, terfenadine, midazolam, cyclosporin, cisapride, quinidine, atorvastatin, simvastatin, lovastatin) can be increased when coadministered with itraconazole. Vice versa, plasma concentrations of itraconazole may become elevated when it is administered concomitantly with other CYP3A4 inhibitors, potentiating its therapeutic and adverse effects. Itraconazole may also increase plasma concentrations of digoxin leading to digitalis toxicity [26,27]. On the other hand, CYP3A4 inducers may decrease the concentrations of itraconazole (eg, phenytoin, rifampin, and isoniazid) (see Table 2) [25,27]. Gastrointestinal absorption of itraconazole from the capsule formulation may be markedly reduced by drugs that increase gastric pH (eg, antacids, H_2 blocker antihistamines, proton pump inhibitors) [26,27].

Ketoconazole

History

Ketoconazole is an imidazole derivative first developed by Janssen Pharmaceutica in 1977 and approved by the FDA in 1981. It is the most widely used and most extensively studied azole antifungal agent [31].

Mechanism

Like other azoles, ketoconazole selectively inhibits fungal cell cytochrome P-450 enzyme 14-α demethylase, inhibiting the conversion of lanosterol to ergosterol required in fungal wall synthesis. It also results in increased permeability of fungal cell membranes. The net result is cessation of fungal cell division and growth. Ketoconazole can also inhibit the synthesis of thromboxane and adrenal steroids such as aldosterone, cortisol, and testosterone by inhibiting cytochrome P-450 enzymes [1,32].

Absorption

Absorption of ketoconazole through the skin is insignificant, with no ketoconazole detected in plasma after topical application of ketoconazole cream or shampooing. Approximately 5% of ketoconazole is found to penetrate into the hair keratin 12 hours after a single shampoo.

Ketoconazole is well absorbed through the gastrointestinal tract. The mean peak plasma levels of ketoconazole reach approximately 3.5 µg/mL within 1 to 2 hours after oral administration of a single 200-mg dose when it is taken with a meal. It is mainly excreted through the bile into the intestinal tract [33].

Available forms

Ketoconazole is available in a cream, shampoo, and tablets.

Pregnancy category

Both topical and oral ketoconazole are rated pregnancy category C.

Clinical indications

Ketoconazole is a broad-spectrum synthetic imidazole antifungal agent that inhibits the growth of dermatophytes and yeasts including *Trichophyton rubrum, T mentagrophytes, T tonsurans, Microsporum canis, M audouini, M gypseum, Epidermophyton floccosum, Candida albicans, C tropicalis, Malassezia ovale*, and *M furfur*. Clinically, ketoconazole cream is effective in the topical treatment of cutaneous candidiasis, tinea manuum, tinea pedis, tinea cruris, and tinea corporis; however, an oral antifungal agent may be added if the disease is extensive. Ketoconazole cream and shampoo are also widely used in the treatment of seborrheic dermatitis because of its activity against *M furfur* [34,35].

Ketoconazole tablets are indicated for the treatment of severe, recalcitrant, cutaneous dermatophyte infections in patients who fail topical therapy or oral griseofulvin, or who are unable to take griseofulvin. Ketoconazole tablets are also indicated for the treatment of systemic fungal infections including candidiasis, chronic mucocutaneous candidiasis, oral thrush, candiduria, blastomycosis, coccidioidomycosis, histoplasmosis, chromomycosis, and paracoccidioidomycosis [33,36]. An off-label use for oral ketoconazole is the treatment of tinea versicolor [36].

Adverse effects

Ketoconazole cream is generally well tolerated by most patients. In clinical trials, common adverse effects such as irritation, pruritus, and stinging have been reported in 3% to 5% of patients receiving ketoconazole 2% cream. Among 905 patients treated with ketoconazole 2% cream, one reported a painful allergic reaction. Rare cases of contact dermatitis have been reported following topical application of ketoconazole cream [35].

The most common adverse effects that have been reported following oral administration of ketoconazole include nausea, vomiting (in approximately 3% of patients), abdominal pain (1.2%), and pruritus (1.5%). Less than 1% of patients may experience headache, dizziness, somnolence, fever, chills, photophobia, diarrhea, gynecomastia, impotence, thrombocytopenia, leukopenia, and hemolytic anemia. Most of these reactions are mild and transient in nature and rarely require discontinuation of ketoconazole. More serious adverse effects such as anaphylaxis, hypersensitivity reactions and hepatic toxicity, suicidal tendencies, and severe depression have been reported in rare cases and warrant special attention and close monitoring [33].

Interactions

Ketoconazole is a potent inhibitor of CYP3A4. The plasma concentrations of drugs primarily metabolized by CYP3A4 (eg, terfenadine, midazolam, cyclosporin, cisapride, quinidine, atorvastatin, simvastatin, lovastatin) can be increased when they are coadministered with ketoconazole. Likewise, the plasma concentrations of ketoconazole may be elevated when it is administered concomitantly with other inhibitors, potentiating its therapeutic and adverse effects. Conversely, CYP3A4 inducers may decrease the concentration of ketoconazole (eg, phenytoin, rifampin, isoniazid) (see Table 2) [25]. Gastrointestinal absorption of ketoconazole from the tablet formulation may be markedly reduced by drugs that increase gastric pH (eg, antacids, H_2 blocker antihistamines, proton pump inhibitors) [33,36].

Miconazole

History

Miconazole, a member of the imidazole antifungal family, is a synthetic 1-phenethylimidazole derivative. It was synthesized in 1969 and later approved by the FDA in 1974 [18].

Mechanism

Like other azoles, miconazole interacts with 14-α demethylase and inhibits the biosynthesis of ergosterol. Subsequent changes in the composition of the lipid components in the fungal cell membrane result in impaired fungal cell division [1]. Miconazole also inhibits peroxidases, which results in the accumulation of peroxide within the cell, resulting in cell death [1,37].

Absorption

Miconazole is poorly soluble in water. Systemic absorption is insignificant with less than 1% of the drug absorbed after topical application; however, miconazole has good penetration to stratum corneum following topical application to skin [4].

Available forms

Miconazole is available as a cream (2%), gel (2%), and vaginal suppositories (100 mg, 200 mg).

Pregnancy category

Miconazole is rated pregnancy category B.

Clinical indications

Topical application of miconazole cream is effective in the treatment of tinea pedis, tinea cruris, and tinea corporis caused by *Trichophyton rubrum*, *T mentagrophytes*, and *Epidermophyton floccosum*. Given its activity against *Candida albicans, C parapsilosis*, and *Malassezia furfur*, miconazole is also used in the treatment of cutaneous candidiasis and tinea versicolor [38]. Miconazole has also shown activity against some gram-positive cocci [38]; however, because of its modest effects, miconazole is not indicated as a first-line therapy in the treatment of such infections.

Adverse effects

There have been isolated reports of irritation, burning, maceration, and allergic contact dermatitis associated with the application of miconazole. Occurrence of cross-sensitivity has been reported among the imidazole-derivative azole antifungals such as clotrimazole, econazole, miconazole, oxiconazole, sulconazole, and tioconazole. The cross-sensitivity appears to be unpredictable [39].

Oxiconazole

History

Oxiconazole, 1-(2,4-dichlorophenyl)-N-[(2,4-dichlorophenyl)methoxy]-2-imidazol-1-yl-ethanimine, is an imidazole derivative. It was first approved by the FDA in 1989 for the topical treatment of dermatomycosis.

Mechanism

Like other azoles, oxiconazole operates its antifungal activity through the inhibition of ergosterol biosynthesis, which is critical for fungal cell membrane integrity.

Absorption

In vitro assays have demonstrated that oxiconazole penetrates well into the skin after topical application. Systemic absorption of oxiconazole following topical application is low.

Available forms

Oxiconazole is available as a cream (1%) and lotion (1%).

Pregnancy category

Oxiconazole is rated pregnancy category B.

Clinical indications

Oxiconazole has fungicidal or fungistatic activity in vitro against *Trichophyton rubrum*, *T mentagrophytes*, *T tonsurans*, *T violaceum*, *Epidermophyton floccosum*, *Microsporum canis*, *M audouini*, *M gypseum*, *Candida albicans*, and *Malassezia furfur*. Oxiconazole appears to be less effective than miconazole and ketoconazole against *Candida albicans* and *C parapsilosis*, respectively. Clinically, topical application of once to twice daily oxiconazole is effective for the treatment of tinea pedis, tinea corporis, or tinea cruris [40]. Once daily application is indicated in the treatment of tinea versicolor [41].

Adverse effects

Most patients tolerate oxiconazole well. Only 2.6% to 4.3% of patients reported adverse reactions during clinical trials. Common adverse effects of topical oxiconazole include pruritus, burning, irritation, stinging, erythema, papules, fissure, maceration, skin eruption, and allergic contact dermatitis [41].

Voriconazole

History

Voriconazole, a newer member of the triazole family, is structurally similar to fluconazole. It differs from fluconazole by replacing a triazole moiety with a fluoropyridine group and adding a methyl group to the propyl backbone. Voriconazole was approved for the treatment of serious fungal infection by the FDA in 2001.

Mechanism

Like other azoles, voriconazole binds and inhibits ergosterol synthesis by inhibiting P-450–dependent lanosterol 14-α demethylase. Depletion of ergosterol and accumulation of lanosterol impair the function and integrity of fungal cell membrane [1].

Absorption

There is no significant difference in the pharmacokinetic properties when voriconazole is administered via intravenous or oral routes. The oral bioavailability of voriconazole is estimated to be 96% based on a population pharmacokinetic analysis of pooled data in 207 healthy subjects. Maximum plasma concentrations (C_{max}) are achieved 1 to 2 hours after the administration of voriconazole. Unlike itraconazole (capsule formulation) and ketoconazole, the absorption of voriconazole is not affected by an increase in gastric pH [42].

Available forms

Voriconazole is available in a film-coated tablet and oral suspension for oral administration and a lyophilized powder for solution for intravenous infusion.

Pregnancy category

Voriconazole is rated pregnancy category D. It can cause fetal harm when administered to a pregnant woman.

Clinical indication

Voriconazole is a broad-spectrum antifungal agent that has shown in vitro activity against *Aspergillus* spp (*A flavus*, *A niger*, *A terreus*, as well as itraconazole and amphotericin B resistant *A fumigatus*,), *Candida* spp (*C glabrata*, *C parapsilosis*, *C tropicalis*, and fluconazole resistant *C albican* and *C krusei*,), *Scedosporium* spp, and *Fusarium* spp [43]. Clinically, voriconazole has been used for serious fungal infections in patients refractory to amphotericin B or other azoles, such as esophageal candidiasis, candidemia, invasive aspergillosis, and fungal infections caused by *Scedosporium apiospermum* and *Fusarium* spp, including *F solani* [44].

Adverse effects

The most common adverse effects of voriconazole include visual disturbances, fever, nausea, vomiting, diarrhea, headache, sepsis, peripheral edema, abdominal pain, and respiratory disorders. Elevated liver function tests may lead to discontinuation of therapy [42]. During clinical trials, approximately 7% of the patients treated with voriconazole reported a skin eruption. Less commonly, photosensitivity reactions can occur with long-term voriconazole treatment. Stevens-Johnson syndrome and toxic epidermal necrolysis are reported rarely [45].

Interactions

Voriconazole undergoes metabolism through the hepatic CYP450 enzyme system mediated by CYP3A4, CYP2C19, and, to a less extent, CYP2C9. Inhibitors of CYP3A4, CYP2C19, or CYP2C9 may increase the plasma concentrations of voriconazole (eg, erythromycin, indinavir, ranitidine and cimetidine, and omeprazole). Conversely, the inducers may decrease the concentrations of voriconazole (eg, phenytoin, rifampicin, rifabutin, St. John's wort). Likewise, voriconazole can alter the plasma concentrations of certain drugs that metabolize via the CYP450 enzyme system, such as cyclosporine, tacrolimus, sirolimus, cyclosporin, wafarin, and phenytoin (see Table 2) [42,46].

Ciclopirox olamine

Ciclopirox is a synthetic hydroxypyridone derivative that carries antifungal, antibacterial, and anti-inflammatory properties. It has a chemical formula of 6-cyclohexyl-1-hydroxy-4-methyl-2[1H]-pyridone. It has been widely used as a topical treatment for superficial fungal infections.

Mechanism

Unlike other antifungals such as azoles and allylamines that act by affecting sterol synthesis, ciclopirox has high affinity for trivalent cations, such as Fe^{3+} and Al^{3+} [47]. By creating a large polyvalent cation through chelation, it inhibits essential enzymes, including cytochromes, interfering with mitochondrial electron transport processes and energy production. Ciclopirox also inhibits cellular uptake of essential compounds and impairs fungi cell membrane integrity at high concentrations and cell respiratory processes. Its anti-inflammatory property is most likely due to inhibition of 5-lipoxygenase and cyclooxygenase and inhibition of prostaglandin and leukotriene [48].

Absorption

Ciclopirox olamine penetrates skin rapidly following topical application. In one in vitro porcine model, a near complete inhibition of *Trichophyton mentagrophytes* growth was achieved in the lower layer of the stratum corneum after application of ciclopirox for 1 hour or longer [49]. Ciclopirox also has good penetration into hair and sebaceous glands through the epidermis and hair follicles. Systemic absorption is minimal, with only 1.3% of the dose absorbed after topical application of 1% ciclopirox cream to the back with occlusion for 6 hours [50].

Available forms

Ciclopirox is available in multiple formulations, including a cream (1%), lotion (1%), gel (0.77% in a free acid form), topical suspension, and nail lacquer (8%).

Pregnancy category

Ciclopirox is rated pregnancy category B.

Clinical indication

Ciclopirox has broad-spectrum fungistatic or fungicidal activity in vitro against dermatophytes (*Trichophyton* spp, *Microsporum* spp, *Epidermatophyton floccosum*), yeasts (*Candida* spp, *Malassezia* spp, *Cryptococcus neoformans*), dimorphic fungi (*Blastomyces dermatitidis*, *Histoplasma capsulatum*), eumycetes, actinomycetes, and various other fungi including *Aspergillus* spp, *Penicillium* spp, *Phialophora* spp, and *Fusarium* spp. Ciclopirox showed greater fungicidal activity against *Trichophyton mentagrophytes* than naftifine and oxiconazole cream in a study conducted by Aly and colleagues [49]. Clinically, ciclopirox 1% cream, lotion, and 0.77% topical suspension are indicated for the treatment of cutaneous candidiasis owing to *Candida albicans*, dermatophytosis such as tinea pedis, tinea cruris, and tinea corporis caused by *Trichophyton rubrum, T mentagrophytes, Epidermatophtyon floccosum,* and *Microsporum canis.* Ciclopirox 0.77% gel is indicated for the topical treatment of seborrheic dermatitis associated with *Malassezia furfur,* interdigital tinea pedis, and tinea corporis. In a clinical trial that compared ciclopirox and clotrimazole cream in the treatment of dermatophyte infections, both agents demonstrated an equivalent cure rate clinically and mycologically, with a more rapid onset of effects when treated with ciclopirox [51]. Ciclopirox lacquer is also used in immunocompetent patients with mild-to-moderate onychomycosis of fingernails and toenails without lunula involvement owing to *Trichophyton rubrum*. Ciclopirox also exhibits antibacterial activity against gram-positive and gram-negative bacteria. It may be an effective agent in treating interdigital tinea pedis with secondary bacterial overgrowth (dermatophytosis complex) [48].

Adverse effects

Adverse effects are rare when ciclopirox is used topically for the treatment of superficial fungal infections. Less than 5% of patients experience side effects in most studies. The most common side effects include irritation, a burning sensation, pain, redness, or pruritus [52].

Griseofulvin

History

Griseofulvin is a metabolic product of *Penicillium griseofulvum* isolated from culture in 1939 by Oxford and colleagues [53]. It is one of the classic oral antifungal agents used for the treatment of dermatophytoses for more than 40 years.

Mechanism

Griseofulvin is fungistatic. Although the exact mechanism by which it inhibits the growth of dermatophytes is unclear, it is thought to act by inhibiting fungal cell mitosis and nuclear acid synthesis, and by interfering with the function of spindle and cytoplasmic microtubules by binding to alpha and beta tubulin [1].

Absorption

Griseofulvin is poorly absorbed from the gastrointestinal tract, with absorption rates ranging from 25% to 70% of an oral dose. Its absorption is significantly enhanced by a fatty meal. The peak plasma concentration occurs about 4 hours after oral administration. It is present in the outer layer of the stratum corneum shortly after it is ingested. Deposition in the keratin precursor cells and a greater affinity for diseased tissue may contribute to its delivery to nails and hair, although the exact mechanism is not known.

Available forms

Griseofulvin is available in capsules, tablets, and oral suspensions.

Pregnancy category

Griseofulvin is in FDA pregnancy category C.

Clinical indication

Griseofulvin is fungistatic with in vitro activity against *Microsporum* spp, *Epidermophyton* spp, and *Trichophyton* spp. It has been used for the treatment of dermatophytosis, including tinea corporis, tinea pedis, tinea cruris, and tinea barbae. For many years, griseofulvin has been the treatment of choice for tinea capitis. The standard doses of 15 to 20 mg/kg/day (microsized form) for 6 to 8 weeks in children have shown cure rates of 64% to 96% [54]. Studies with newer antifungal agents such as terbinafine and itraconazole have shown encouraging results; however, terbinafine is not as effective against *Microsporum canis* infection [55]. Griseofulvin has also been used in the treatment of onychomycosis caused by dermatophytes; however, due to its long treatment period from 6 to 18 months, many relapses, and disappointing results, newer oral antifungals such as terbinafine are preferred in treating onychomycosis.

Adverse effects

Griseofulvin is well tolerated in most patients, especially in children. Most adverse effects are minor, including headaches, gastrointestinal reactions, and cutaneous eruptions [56].

Interactions

Griseofulvin may potentially cause loss of efficacy of oral contraceptives, an increased incidence of breakthrough bleeding, and menstrual irregularities [57]. With coadministration of griseofulvin, patients who are on warfarin-type anticoagulants may require dose adjustment of the anticoagulant during and after griseofulvin therapy. Concomitant use of barbiturates may depress griseofulvin activity [56].

Allylamines and benzylamines

The allylamines were introduced in 1980s as agents that exhibited a broader spectrum of fungicidal activity against dermatophytes such as *Trichophyton rubrum*, *T mentagrophytes*, *T tonsurans*, and *Epidermophyton floccosum*. *Microsporum canis*, *M audouini*, and *M gypseum* are relatively more resistant to allylamines. Allylamines are also fungistatic against *Candida* spp. They work through a common mode of action by inhibiting squalene epoxidase, which is an essential enzyme in the ergosterol biosynthesis pathway of fungal cell membrane formation. They are selective for fungal enzymes and have little effect on mammalian cholesterol synthesis [58]. The two main antimycotics in the allylamines family are terbinafine and naftifine. Benzylamines are another class of antifungals that are structurally similar to the allylamines. They operate via a similar mode of action by blocking the epoxidation of squalene. Butenafine is the representative drug in this class.

Naftifine

History

Naftifine is a synthetic allylamine derivative that was incidentally discovered from research into new agents for the treatment of central nervous system disorders. It carries a chemical name of (E)-N-cinnamyl-N-methyl-1-naphthalenemethyl-amine-3-phenyl-2-propen-1-amine hydrochloride.

Mechanism

Naftifine interferes with biosynthesis of ergosterol by inhibiting the enzyme squalene 2,3-epoxidase that converts squalene to squalene oxide. This inhibition of enzyme activity leads to decreased amounts of ergosterol and an accumulation of squalene in the cells and disruption of fungal cell membrane [59].

Absorption

Systemic absorption of naftifine is approximately 6% of the applied dose after a single topical application. Naftifine is highly lipophilic, allowing for good penetration into the stratum corneum and hair follicles.

Available forms

Naftifine is available in a cream (1%) and gel (1%) formulation.

Pregnancy category

Naftifine is rated pregnancy category B.

Clinical indication

Naftifine is a broad-spectrum allylamine derivative that exhibits fungicidal activity in vitro against *Trichophyton rubrum*, *T mentagrophytes*, *T tonsurans*, *Epidermophyton floccosum*, and *Microsporum* spp, and fungistatic activity against *Candida* spp. Clinically, it is indicated for the topical treatment of tinea pedis, tinea cruris, and tinea corporis due to *Trichophyton rubrum*, *T mentagrophytes*, *T tonsurans*, and *Epidermophyton floccosum* [60]. Naftifine achieved equivalent effects with an earlier onset of action in the treatment of tinea cruris and tinea corporis when compared with econazole cream in a controlled double-blind study [61]. It is also effective in the treatment of cutaneous candidiasis.

Adverse effects

Adverse effects are minor. The most common side effects of naftifine include burning, stinging, dryness, erythema, itching, local irritation, and, rarely, allergic reactions (data on file, Herbert Laboratories, Irvine, California, 1985).

Terbinafine

History

Terbinafine is a synthetic allylamine antifungal agent that has a chemical name of (E)-N-(6,6-dimethyl-2-hepten-4-ynyl)-N-methyl-1-naphthalene-methanamine hydrochloride. It was developed in 1979 with chemical modification of naftifine.

Mechanism

Terbinafine acts by inhibiting the membrane-bound squalene epoxidase, interrupting the conversion of squalene to squalene oxide. It blocks the biosynthesis of ergosterol, impairing fungal cellular integrity. The intracellular accumulation of squalene results in fungal cell death [59,62].

Absorption

Systemic absorption of terbinafine is clinically insignificant. Only 3% to 5% of the applied dosage is absorbed systemically following topical application of 1% terbinafine cream. Terbinafine is well absorbed from the gastrointestinal tract after oral administration, with the peak plasma concentration of 1 µg/mL detected within 2 hours after a single 250-mg dose [63]. Because terbinafine is highly lipophilic, it accumulates in the stratum corneum, sebum, and hair follicles efficiently. Terbinafine can be detected in the stratum corneum 24 hours after oral administration. It is also detected in the hair and distal nails within

1 week of starting therapy at a dose of 250 mg/day [64].

Pregnancy category

Topical terbinafine is rated pregnancy category B. Oral terbinafine is in pregnancy category B.

Clinical indication

Terbinafine has demonstrated excellent in vitro fungicidal activity against various dermatophytes, including *Tricophyton mentagrophytes, T rubrum, T tonsurans,* and *Epidermophyton floccosum.* It also exhibits potent activity against *Candida* spp, including *C albicans* and *C parapsilosis,* nondermatophyte molds such as *Scopulariopsis* spp, and *Aspergillus* spp [65,66]. Topical application of terbinafine 1% cream has been shown to be effective in the treatment of tinea cruris, tinea corporis, pityriasis versicolor, and intertriginous candidiasis in a multicenter study of 629 patients in Japan [67]. Once or twice daily topical application of terbinafine 1% cream for up to 2 weeks achieved mycologic cure in greater than 80% of patients with tinea pedis, tinea corporis, tinea cruris, cutaneous candidiasis, and pityriasis versicolor. It is as effective as topical miconazole and naftifine in tinea pedis and more effective than clotrimazole and oxiconazole [68–70]. In another clinical study, topical application of terbinafine 1% cream achieved mycologic eradication and clinical improvement of tinea corporis and tinea cruris in 76% of patients. Only 17% of patients receiving placebo achieved similar results [71].

Terbinafine tablets are approved by the FDA for the treatment of onychomycosis of the toenail or fingernail due to dermatophytes. The recommended dose is 250 mg/day for 6 weeks for fingernail onychomycosis and for 12 weeks in the treatment of toenail onychomycosis [72]. Off-label uses of terbinafine include the treatment of onychomycosis in children, onychomycosis due to *Candida* spp, and some nondermatophyte molds, tinea cruris, tinea pedis, tinea corporis, and tinea capitis [73]. Terbinafine may not be as effective in treating tinea capitis caused by ectothrix infections such as *Microsporum canis,* which may require a longer duration of treatment.

Adverse effects

Terbinafine tablets are well tolerated in general. The most frequently reported adverse events are mild and transient, including gastrointestinal symptoms (eg, diarrhea, dyspepsia, abdominal pain), liver function test abnormalities, rashes, urticaria, pruritus, and taste disturbances. Because hepatotoxicity may occur rarely in patients with and without preexisting liver disease, liver function should be tested before starting therapy. Infrequently, precipitation and exacerbation of cutaneous and systemic lupus erythematosus and, rarely, a severe rash including erythema multiforme have been reported (data on file, Novartis Pharma AG, Basel, Switzerland, 1997). Adverse effects of topical terbinafine cream are mostly mild and localized to the application site, including burning, tingling, dryness, and pruritus [74].

Interactions

Terbinafine undergoes extensive metabolism in the liver. When compared with azoles, terbinafine has affinity for less than 5% of CYP enzymes, giving it a relatively low potential for affecting the metabolism of other drugs. Nevertheless, terbinafine is a potent inhibitor of CYP2D6 and affects drugs that are predominantly metabolized by this enzyme, such as tricyclic antidepressants, β-blockers, some selective serotonin reuptake inhibitors, and monoamine oxidase inhibitors type B. Terbinafine decreases the clearance of caffeine by 19% and increases the clearance of cyclosporine by 15%. CYP450 inducers such as rifampin increase the clearance of terbinafine, and CYP450 inhibitors such as cimetidine decrease the clearance of terbinafine [75]. Terbinafine does not inhibit the metabolism of tolbutamide, ethinylestradiol, ethoxycoumarin, and cyclosporine in in vitro studies. In vivo drug-drug interaction studies have shown that the clearance of antipyrine or digoxin in healthy volunteers is not affected by terbinafine [75].

Butenafine

Butenafine is a representative benzylamine derivative with a chemical structure and mode of action similar to allylamines. Butenafine has a chemical name of *N*-(4-*tert*-butylbenzyl)-*N*-methyl-1-naphthalenemethylamine hydrochloride.

Mechanism

Like allylamines, butenafine inhibits the membrane-bound squalene epoxidase, interrupting the conversion of squalene to squalene oxide, which results in intracellular accumulation of squalene. It blocks the biosynthesis of ergosterol, resulting in increased cellular permeability, leakage of cellular contents, and fungal cell death [59].

Absorption

Systemic absorption of butenafine cream through the skin is low. The mean plasma concentration of butenafine was 0.91 µg/L following a once-daily topical application of butenafine 1% cream in patients with tinea cruris for 14 days [76].

Clinical indication

Butenafine exhibits excellent fungicidal activity in vitro and in animal models against dermatophytes, dimorphic fungi, and *Aspergillus* spp, with a greater mycologic eradication when compared with that of terbinafine, naftifine, and clotrimazole [77]. It is also active against *Candida albicans*, and its activity is superior to that of terbinafine and naftifine [78]. Clinically, once daily application of butenafine cream has been used for the topical treatment of tinea versicolor due to *Malassezia furfur*, interdigital tinea pedis, tinea corporis, and tinea cruris caused by dermatophytes such as *Epidermophyton floccosum*, *Trichophyton mentagrophytes*, *T rubrum*, and *T tonsurans*.

Available forms

Butenafine is available in a cream (1%) formulation.

Adverse effects

Adverse effects of butenafine are mild. Only 1% of patients treated with butenafine 1% cream in controlled clinical trials report adverse events, including burning, stinging, and an itching sensation at the site of application. Other reported adverse effects occurring in less than 2% of patients include contact dermatitis, erythema, and skin irritation [74,79].

Echinocandins

The echinocandins are a new class of antifungal drug that have significantly expanded the options for treatment of invasive fungal infections. They have potent fungicidal activity against various *Candida* spp, including *C albicans, C glabrata, C dubliniensis, C tropicalis, C krusei, C parapsilosis,* and *C guilliermondii.* They are also effective against *Aspergillus* spp, including *A fumigatus, A flavus,* and *A terreus.* Echinocandins exert their antifungal action through noncompetitive inhibition of the synthesis of 1,3-β-glucans, an essential component of the fungal cell wall [1,80]. They appear to be highly effective even against azole resistant fungi. The echinocandins are not metabolized through the hepatic CYP450 enzyme

system, with the benefit of fewer drug interactions when compared with azoles. The FDA has approved caspofungin, followed by micafungin and most recently anidulafungin, for the treatment of esophageal candidiasis and candidemia. This review focuses on caspofungin and micafungin.

Caspofungin

History

Caspofungin, the first approved echinocandin, is a semisynthetic derivative of the pneumocandin B_0, a fermentation product of the fungus *Glarea lozoyensis*. Caspofungin received FDA approval in 2001.

Mechanism

Caspofungin acts through inhibition of the synthesis of β-(1,3)-D-glucan, an essential component of the cell wall of *Candida* and *Aspergillus* spp that is not present in mammalian cells.

Absorption

Caspofungin is not absorbed when administered orally; therefore, the drug is administered by slow intravenous infusion. The mean peak plasma concentrations are 7.6 and 12.3 µg/mL, respectively, after single doses of 50 and 70 mg. The plasma clearance of caspofungin is determined by the rate of distribution from plasma to tissue rather than by the rate of metabolism or excretion [81]. Because it is highly protein bound, 92% tissue distribution is achieved within 36 to 48 hours following intravenous infusion.

Available forms

Caspofungin is available in a lyophilized powder for solution administered via intravenous infusion.

Pregnancy category

Caspofungin is rated pregnancy category C.

Clinical indication

Caspofungin has demonstrated excellent in vitro activity against *Aspergillus* spp, including *A fumigatus*, *A flavus*, and *A terreus*, and *Candida* spp, including *C albicans, C glabrata, C guilliermondii, C krusei, C parapsilosis,* and *C tropicalis* [82,83]. In a double-blind, randomized comparison study in 224 patients with invasive candidiasis and candidemia, the response rates were 73% for caspofungin and 62% for amphotericin B. Caspofungin was given at a loading dose of 70 mg on day 1 followed by a maintenance dose of 50 mg/day, and amphotericin B deoxycholate was given at a dose of either 0.6 or 1 mg/kg/day (depending on the status of neutropenia). In patients who had received therapy for at least 5 days, the response rate of caspofungin (81%) was superior to that of amphotericin B (65%). The tolerability was also significantly superior in the caspofungin-treated group [84]. Caspofungin is approved by the FDA for the treatment of esophageal candidiasis and candidemia, for salvage therapy of *Aspergillus* spp infections, and for empirical therapy in neutropenic patients with refractory fever.

Adverse effects

Caspofungin is generally well tolerated. The most common adverse effects after a loading dose of 70 mg followed by a daily maintenance dose of 50 mg include fever, chills, headache, phlebitis/thrombophlebitis, nausea, vomiting, abdominal pain, diarrhea, and skin eruption or flushing. Serious adverse events such as anaphylaxis and pulmonary infiltrates may rarely occur. The most common laboratory abnormalities reported include hypokalemia, hypoalbuminemia, elevated ALT, AST, or alkaline phosphatase, decreased hemoglobin, increased urinary protein, hypercalcemia, leukopenia, and elevated creatinine [85,86]. The elevation of transaminases is usually transient and modest with no clinical evidence of hepatotoxicity.

Interactions

Caspofungin is metabolized via hydrolysis and N-acetylation. It does not inhibit or induce the CYP450 enzyme system; therefore, fewer drug interactions are expected when this agent is compared with azole antifungals. The pharmacokinetics of caspofungin are not changed by itraconazole, amphotericin B, mycophenolate, nelfinavir, or tacrolimus in clinical studies. Caspofungin has no effect on the pharmacokinetics of itraconazole, amphotericin B, or the active metabolite of mycophenolate [87]. Coadministration of tacrolimus with caspofungin was reported to reduce the area under the curve (AUC) of tacrolimus by approximately 20% to 40% and C_{max} by 16%. Appropriate monitoring of tacrolimus blood concentrations and adjustments of tacrolimus dosage may be necessary in patients receiving both therapies. Cyclosporine can increase the AUC of caspofungin while caspofungin does not alter the plasma levels of cyclosporine. Coadministration of rifampin, efavirenz, nevirapine, phenytoin, dexamethasone, or carbamazepine with caspofungin can decrease the plasma concentration of caspofungin [88].

Micafungin

History

Micafungin, a member of the echinocandin class, is a semisynthetic lipopeptide synthesized from a fermentation product of the fungus *Coleophoma empetri*. The FDA approved it for use in clinical practice in 2005.

Mechanism

Like other echinocadins, micafungin blocks 1,3-β-D-glucan synthase, inhibiting the synthesis of 1,3-β-D-glucan, a critical component of fungal cell wall, resulting in osmotic disruption of the fungal cell.

Absorption

Like caspofungin, micafungin is absorbed poorly when administered orally; therefore, it is administered through intravenous infusion. The AUC and C_{max} of micafungin appear to be of relative dose proportionality [89]. The maximum plasma concentration of 4.9 mg/L was achieved following intravenous infusion of micafungin at a dose of 50 mg in healthy volunteers. The elimination half-life ranged from 11 to 15 hours [90].

Available forms

Micafungin is available as a lyophilized powder for solution for intravenous infusion.

Pregnancy category

Micafungin is rated pregnancy category C.

Clinical indication

Micafungin shares with caspofungin a same spectrum of in vitro activity against *Candida* spp, *Aspergillus* spp, and several molds. It is indicated for the treatment of esophageal candidiasis and for prophylaxis of *Candida* infection in patients undergoing hematopoietic stem cell transplantation. In a nonblind multinational trial, 88% of patients (60 of 68) with newly diagnosed candidemia and 76% (39 of 51) of patients with refractory candidemia receiving micafungin therapy achieved a complete or partial response. The mean duration of treatment was 20 days [91]. In another multicenter trial to evaluate the efficacy of micafungin in the treatment of patients with presumed aspergillosis or candidiasis, a mycologic cure was achieved in 63% (12 of 19) of patients with infections caused by *Aspergillus flavus, A fumigatus, A niger*, or *A terreus* and in 50% (4 of 8) of patients infected with *Candida albicans, C glabrata*, or *C krusei* [92].

Adverse effects

The most commonly reported side effects of micafungin include nausea, vomiting, and elevated liver function tests. Possible histamine-mediated symptoms such as skin eruption, pruritus, facial swelling, and vasodilatation have been reported with micafungin, but not as frequently as with caspofungin. Phlebitis and thrombophlebitis at the injection site have also been reported [93].

Interactions

Studies have been conducted to evaluate the potential for interaction between micafungin and mycophenolate mofetil, cyclosporine, tacrolimus, prednisolone, sirolimus, nifedipine, fluconazole, ritonavir, and rifampin. The pharmacokinetics of micafungin were not altered by these drugs. Likewise, micafungin demonstrated no effects on the pharmacokinetics of mycophenolate mofetil, cyclosporine, tacrolimus, prednisolone, and fluconazole. The AUC of sirolimus and the AUC and C_{max} of nifedipine were increased when administered with micafungin concomitantly (data on file, Fujisawa Healthcare, Deerfield, Illinois, 2005).

Summary

Until the 1940s, choices of antifungal agents were limited for the treatment of superficial and invasive fungal infections. In the past several decades, development of the polyene and azole antifungals has been a milestone in the history of medical mycology. Nevertheless, their associated adverse effects, drug-drug interactions, the emergence of resistance, and the increased incidence of opportunistic fungal infections in immunocompromised patients urged the development of newer generations of antifungal agents. The development of allylamine and benzylamine antifungals represented a major success. With their fungicidal activity against dermatophytes, they have been widely used in the treatment of cutaneous dermatophytosis and onychomycosis.

The second generation of triazoles, such as voriconazole, lipid formulation of the polyenes, and a new class of antifungal agents, the echinocandins, have demonstrated a broadened spectrum of antifungal activities, better efficacy, an improved safety profile, and less drug-drug interactions. They have also shown great therapeutic and prophylactic benefit in the battle against pathogenic fungi. This review has focused on the advances of these newer antifungal agents. Even newer antifungals, including posaconazole, ravuconazole, and anidulafungin, are on the horizon and have shown promise in clinical results, yet the search for ideal antifungal agents continues.

References

[1] Georgopapadakou NH. Antifungals: mechanism of action and resistance, established and novel drugs. Curr Opin Microbiol 1998;1(5):547–57.

[2] Hazen EL, Brown R. Two antifungal agents produced by a soil actinomycete. Science 1950; 112(2911):423.

[3] Hazen EL, Brown R. Nystatin. Ann N Y Acad Sci 1960;89:258–66.

[4] Bennett JE. Antimicrobial agents: antifungal agents. In: Gilaman AG, Nies AS, editors. The pharmacological basis of therapeutics. New York: McGraw-Hill; 1993. p. 1165–81.

[5] Kuriyama T, Williams DW, Bagg J, et al. In vitro susceptibility of oral *Candida* to seven antifungal agents. Oral Microbiol Immunol 2005;20(6):349–53.

[6] Wasilewski C Jr. Allergic contact dermatitis from nystatin. Arch Dermatol 1970;102(2):216–7.

[7] Garty BZ. Stevens-Johnson syndrome associated with nystatin treatment. Arch Dermatol 1991; 127(5):741–2.

[8] Epstein JB, Truelove EL, Hanson-Huggins K, et al. Topical polyene antifungals in hematopoietic cell transplant patients: tolerability and efficacy. Support Care Cancer 2004;12(7):517–25.

[9] Gold W, Stout HA, Pagano JF, et al. Amphotericins A and B, antifungal anitbiotics produced by streptomycete I in vitro studies. Antibiotics Ann 1955;3: 579–86.

[10] Ng AW, Wasan KM, Lopez-Berestein G. Development of liposomal polyene antibiotics: an historical perspective. J Pharm Pharm Sci 2003;6(1):67 83.

[11] Ellis D. Amphotericin B: spectrum and resistance. J Antimicrob Chemother 2002;49(Suppl 1):7–10.

[12] Girois SB, Chapuis F, Decullier E, et al. Adverse effects of antifungal therapies in invasive fungal infections: review and meta-analysis. Eur J Clin Microbiol Infect Dis 2006;25(2):138–49.

[13] Kleinberg M. What is the current and future status of conventional amphotericin B? Int J Antimicrob Agents 2006;27(Suppl 1):12–6.

[14] Buchel KH, Draber W, Regel E, et al. Synthesis and properties of clotrimazole and other antimycotic 1-triphenylmethylimidazoles. Arzneimittelforschung 1972;22(8):1260–72.

[15] Holt RJ, Newman RL. Laboratory assessment of the antimycotic drug clotrimazole. J Clin Pathol 1972;25(12):1089–97.

[16] Clayton YM, Connor BL. Comparison of clotrimazole cream, Whitfield's ointment and nystatin ointment for the topical treatment of ringworm

infections, pityriasis versicolor, erythrasma and candidiasis. Br J Dermatol 1973;89(3):297–303.

[17] Rajan VS, Thirumoorthy T. Treatment of cutaneous candidiasis: a double blind, parallel comparison of sulconazole nitrate 1% cream and clotrimazole 1% cream. Australas J Dermatol 1983;24(1):33–6.

[18] Godefroi EF, Heeres J, Van Cutsem J, et al. The preparation and antimycotic properties of derivatives of 1-phenethylimidazole. J Med Chem 1969; 12(5):784–91.

[19] Heel RC, Brogden RN, Speight TM, et al. Econazole: a review of its antifungal activity and therapeutic efficacy. Drugs 1978;16(3):177–201.

[20] Bigardi AS, Pigatto PD, Altomare G. Allergic contact dermatitis due to sulconazole. Contact Dermatitis 1992;26(4):281–2.

[21] Grant SM, Clissold SP. Fluconazole: a review of its pharmacodynamic and pharmacokinetic properties, and therapeutic potential in superficial and systemic mycoses. Drugs 1990;39(6):877–916.

[22] Fluconazole [package insert]. New York: Pfizer Roerig; 1997.

[23] Pham CP, de Feiter PW, van der Kuy PH, et al. Long QTc interval and torsade de pointes caused by fluconazole. Ann Pharmacother 2006;40(7–8): 1456–61.

[24] Gussenhoven MJ, Haak A, Peereboom-Wynia JD, et al. Stevens-Johnson syndrome after fluconazole. Lancet 1991;338(8759):120.

[25] Yu DT, Peterson JF, Seger DL, et al. Frequency of potential azole drug-drug interactions and consequences of potential fluconazole drug interactions. Pharmacoepidemiol Drug Saf 2005;14(11): 755–67.

[26] Gupta AK, Sauder DN, Shear NH. Antifungal agents: an overview. Part II. J Am Acad Dermatol 1994;30(6):911–33 [quiz: 34–6].

[27] Itraconazole [package insert]. Titusville (NJ): Janssen; 1996.

[28] Gupta AK, Sibbald RG, Lynde CW, et al. Onychomycosis in children: prevalence and treatment strategies. J Am Acad Dermatol 1997;36(3 Pt 1): 395–402.

[29] Gupta AK, Alexis ME, Raboobee N, et al. Itraconazole pulse therapy is effective in the treatment of tinea capitis in children: an open multicentre study. Br J Dermatol 1997;137(2):251–4.

[30] Doncker PD, Gupta AK, Marynissen G, et al. Itraconazole pulse therapy for onychomycosis and dermatomycoses: an overview. J Am Acad Dermatol 1997;37(6):969–74.

[31] Heeres J, Backx LJ, Mostmans JH, et al. Antimycotic imidazoles. Part 4. Synthesis and antifungal activity of ketoconazole, a new potent orally active broad-spectrum antifungal agent. J Med Chem 1979;22(8):1003–5.

[32] Mahler C, Verhelst J, Denis L. Ketoconazole and liarozole in the treatment of advanced prostatic cancer. Cancer 1993;71(3 Suppl):1068–73.

[33] Nizoral tablets [package insert]. Titusville (NJ): Janssen Pharmaceutica; 2001.

[34] Odds FC, Milne LJ, Gentles JC, et al. The activity in vitro and in vivo of a new imidazole antifungal, ketoconazole. J Antimicrob Chemother 1980;6(1): 97–104.

[35] Lester M. Ketoconazole 2 percent cream in the treatment of tinea pedis, tinea cruris, and tinea corporis. Cutis 1995;55(3):181–3.

[36] Gupta AK, Sauder DN, Shear NH. Antifungal agents: an overview. Part I. J Am Acad Dermatol 1994;30(5 Pt 1):677–98 [quiz: 698–700].

[37] Fothergill AW. Miconazole: a historical perspective. Expert Rev Anti Infect Ther 2006;4(2):171–5.

[38] Van Cutsem JM, Thienpont D. Miconazole, a broadspectrum antimycotic agent with antibacterial activity. Chemotherapy 1972;17(6):392–404.

[39] Dooms-Goossens A, Matura M, Drieghe J, et al. Contact allergy to imidazoles used as antimycotic agents. Contact Dermatitis 1995;33(2):73–7.

[40] Elewski BE, Jones T, Zaias N. Comparison of an antifungal agent used alone with an antifungal used with a topical steroid in inflammatory tinea pedis. Cutis 1996;58(4):305–7.

[41] Jegasothy BV, Pakes GE. Oxiconazole nitrate: pharmacology, efficacy, and safety of a new imidazole antifungal agent. Clin Ther 1991;13(1):126–41.

[42] Vfend [package insert]. New York: Pfizer Roerig; 2003.

[43] Herbrecht R. Voriconazole: therapeutic review of a new azole antifungal. Expert Rev Anti Infect Ther 2004;2(4):485–97.

[44] Heyn K, Tredup A, Salvenmoser S, et al. Effect of voriconazole combined with micafungin against *Candida, Aspergillus,* and *Scedosporium* spp and *Fusarium solani.* Antimicrob Agents Chemother 2005;49(12):5157–9.

[45] Racette AJ, Roenigk HH Jr, Hansen R, et al. Photoaging and phototoxicity from long-term voriconazole treatment in a 15-year-old girl. J Am Acad Dermatol 2005;52(5 Suppl 1):S81–5.

[46] Boucher HW, Groll AH, Chiou CC, et al. Newer systemic antifungal agents: pharmacokinetics, safety and efficacy. Drugs 2004;64(18):1997–2020.

[47] Korting HC, Grundmann-Kollmann M. The hydroxypyridones: a class of antimycotics of its own. Mycoses 1997;40(7–8):243–7.

[48] Abrams BB, Hanel H, Hoehler T. Ciclopirox olamine: a hydroxypyridone antifungal agent. Clin Dermatol 1991;9(4):471–7.

[49] Aly R, Maibach HI, Bagatell FK, et al. Ciclopirox olamine lotion 1%: bioequivalence to ciclopirox olamine cream 1% and clinical efficacy in tinea pedis. Clin Ther 1989;11(3):290–303.

[50] Ciclopirox olamine. In: Physician's desk reference. Montvale (NJ): Medical Economics Company; 1999. p. 1327.

[51] Bogaert H, Cordero C, Ollague W, et al. Multicentre double-blind clinical trials of ciclopirox olamine

cream 1% in the treatment of tinea corporis and tinea cruris. J Int Med Res 1986;14(4):210–6.

[52] Jue SG, Dawson GW, Brogden RN. Ciclopirox olamine 1% cream: a preliminary review of its antimicrobial activity and therapeutic use. Drugs 1985; 29(4):330–41.

[53] Oxford AE, Raistrick H, Simonart P, et al. Studies in the biochemistry of micro-organisms: Griseofulvin, C(17)H(17)O(6)Cl, a metabolic product of Peincillium griseofulvum Dierckx. Mycoses 2006;49(3): 232–5.

[54] Tanz RR, Hebert AA, Esterly NB. Treating tinea capitis: should ketoconazole replace griseofulvin? J Pediatr 1988;112(6):987–91.

[55] Dragos V, Lunder M. Lack of efficacy of 6-week treatment with oral terbinafine for tinea capitis due to *Microsporum canis* in children. Pediatr Dermatol 1997;14(1):46–8.

[56] Bennett ML, Fleischer AB, Loveless JW, et al. Oral griseofulvin remains the treatment of choice for tinea capitis in children. Pediatr Dermatol 2000;17(4): 304–9.

[57] Cote J. Interaction of griseofulvin and oral contraceptives. J Am Acad Dermatol 1990;22(1):124–5.

[58] Ryder NS, Dupont MC. Inhibition of squalene epoxidase by allylamine antimycotic compounds: a comparative study of the fungal and mammalian enzymes. Biochem J 1985;230(3):765–70.

[59] Ryder NS. Squalene epoxidase as a target for the allylamines. Biochem Soc Trans 1991;19(3):774–7.

[60] Monk JP, Brogden RN. Naftifine: a review of its antimicrobial activity and therapeutic use in superficial dermatomycoses. Drugs 1991;42(4):659–72.

[61] Millikan LE, Galen WK, Gewirtzman GB, et al. Naftifine cream 1% versus econazole cream 1% in the treatment of tinea cruris and tinea corporis. J Am Acad Dermatol 1988;18(1 Pt 1):52–6.

[62] Roberts DT. Oral terbinafine (Lamisil) in the treatment of fungal infections of the skin and nails. Dermatology 1997;194(Suppl 1):37–9.

[63] Kovarik JM, Kirkesseli S, Humbert H, et al. Dose-proportional pharmacokinetics of terbinafine and its N-demethylated metabolite in healthy volunteers. Br J Dermatol 1992;126(Suppl 39):8–13.

[64] Faergemann J, Zehender H, Millerioux L. Levels of terbinafine in plasma, stratum corneum, dermis-epidermis (without stratum corneum), sebum, hair and nails during and after 250 mg terbinafine orally once daily for 7 and 14 days. Clin Exp Dermatol 1994; 19(2):121–6.

[65] Petranyi G, Meingassner JG, Mieth H. Antifungal activity of the allylamine derivative terbinafine in vitro. Antimicrob Agents Chemother 1987;31(9): 1365–8.

[66] Shadomy S, Espinel-Ingroff A, Gebhart RJ. In vitro studies with SF 86-327, a new orally active allylamine derivative. Sabouraudia 1985;23(2): 125–32.

[67] Kagawa S. Clinical efficacy of terbinafine in 629 Japanese patients with dermatomycosis. Clin Exp Dermatol 1989;14(2):114–5.

[68] Bergstresser PR, Elewski B, Hanifin J, et al. Topical terbinafine and clotrimazole in interdigital tinea pedis: a multicenter comparison of cure and relapse rates with 1- and 4-week treatment regimens. J Am Acad Dermatol 1993;28(4):648–51.

[69] Evans EG, Dodman B, Williamson DM, et al. Comparison of terbinafine and clotrimazole in treating tinea pedis. BMJ 1993;307(6905):645–7.

[70] Vermeer BJ, Staats CC, van Houwelingen JC. [Terbinafine versus miconazole in patients with tinea pedis]. Ned Tijdschr Geneeskd 1996;140(31): 1605–8.

[71] Savin RC. Treatment of chronic tinea pedis (athlete's foot type) with topical terbinafine. J Am Acad Dermatol 1990;23(4 Pt 2):786–9.

[72] Alpsoy E, Yilmaz E, Basaran E. Intermittent therapy with terbinafine for dermatophyte toe-onychomycosis: a new approach. J Dermatol 1996;23(4): 259–62.

[73] Tausch I, Decroix J, Gwiezdzinski Z, et al. Short-term itraconazole versus terbinafine in the treatment of tinea pedis or manus. Int J Dermatol 1998;37(2): 140–2.

[74] Villars V, Jones TC. Clinical efficacy and tolerability of terbinafine (Lamisil): a new topical and systemic fungicidal drug for treatment of dermatomycoses. Clin Exp Dermatol 1989;14(2):124–7.

[75] Darkes MJ, Scott LJ, Goa KL. Terbinafine: a review of its use in onychomycosis in adults. Am J Clin Dermatol 2003;4(1):39–65.

[76] Lesher JL Jr, Babel DE, Stewart DM, et al. Butenafine 1% cream in the treatment of tinea cruris: a multicenter, vehicle-controlled, double-blind trial. J Am Acad Dermatol 1997;36(2 Pt 1):S20–4.

[77] Maeda T, Takase M, Ishibashi A, et al. Synthesis and antifungal activity of butenafine hydrochloride (KP-363), a new benzylamine antifungal agent. Yakugaku Zasshi 1991;111(2):126–37.

[78] Syed TA, Maibach HI. Butenafine hydrochloride: for the treatment of interdigital tinea pedis. Expert Opin Pharmacother 2000;1(3):467–73.

[79] Savin R, De Villez RL, Elewski B, et al. One-week therapy with twice-daily butenafine 1% cream versus vehicle in the treatment of tinea pedis: a multicenter, double-blind trial. J Am Acad Dermatol 1997; 36(2 Pt 1):S15–9.

[80] Odds FC, Brown AJ, Gow NA. Antifungal agents: mechanisms of action. Trends Microbiol 2003; 11(6):272–9.

[81] Stone JA, Holland SD, Wickersham PJ, et al. Single- and multiple-dose pharmacokinetics of caspofungin in healthy men. Antimicrob Agents Chemother 2002;46(3):739–45.

[82] Graybill JR, Bocanegra R, Luther M, et al. Treatment of murine *Candida krusei* or *Candida glabrata*

infection with L-743,872. Antimicrob Agents Chemother 1997;41(9):1937–9.

[83] Graybill JR, Najvar LK, Luther MF, et al. Treatment of murine disseminated candidiasis with L-743,872. Antimicrob Agents Chemother 1997;41(8): 1775–7.

[84] Mora-Duarte J, Betts R, Rotstein C, et al. Comparison of caspofungin and amphotericin B for invasive candidiasis. N Engl J Med 2002;347(25):2020–9.

[85] Walsh TJ, Teppler H, Donowitz GR, et al. Caspofungin versus liposomal amphotericin B for empirical antifungal therapy in patients with persistent fever and neutropenia. N Engl J Med 2004;351(14): 1391–402.

[86] Maertens J, Raad I, Petrikkos G, et al. Efficacy and safety of caspofungin for treatment of invasive aspergillosis in patients refractory to or intolerant of conventional antifungal therapy. Clin Infect Dis 2004;39(11):1563–71.

[87] MSD Sharp & Dohme Ltd. Caspofungin MSD: summary of product characteristics. Available at: http://www.eudra.org, 2004.

[88] Maschmeyer G, Glasmacher A. Pharmacological properties and clinical efficacy of a recently licensed systemic antifungal, caspofungin. Mycoses 2005; 48(4):227–34.

[89] Hiemenz J, Simpson D, Devine S, et al. Maximum tolerated dose and pharmacokinetics of FK463 in combination with fluconazole for the prophylaxis of fungal infections in adult bone marrow or peripheral stem cell transplant patients. In: Program and abstracts of the 39th Interscience Conference on Antimicrobial Agents and Chemotherapy [abstract 1648]. San Francisco (CA), September 26–29, 1999.

[90] Mukai T, Nakahara K, Takaya T, et al. Pharmacokinetics of FK463, a novel echinocandin analogue, in elderly and nonelderly subjects. In: Program and abstracts of the 41st Interscience Conference on Antimicrobial Agents and Chemotherapy. Chicago, December 16–19, 2001.

[91] Ostrosky-Zeichner L, Anaissie E, Kontoyiannia D, et al. Micafungin (MCFG), an echinocandin antifungal agent for the treatment of new and refractory candidemia [abstract P-35]. Presented at the 13th Annual Focus on Fungal Infections Meeting. Maui (HI), Mar 19–21, 2003.

[92] Kohno S, Yamaguchi H. A multicenter, open-label clinical study of FK463 in patients with deep mycosis in Japan [abstract]. Presented at the 41st Interscience Conference on Antimicrobial Agents and Chemotherapy. Chicago, Dec 16–19, 2001.

[93] Powles R, Chopra R, et al. Assessment of maximum tolerated dose and pharmacokinetics of FK463 in neutropenic patients after haematopoietic stem cell transplantation [abstract]. Blood 2001; 98(Pt 2):361.

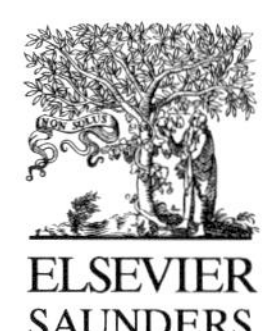

ELSEVIER
SAUNDERS

Dermatol Clin 25 (2007) 185–193

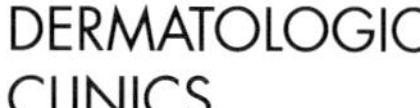

DERMATOLOGIC
CLINICS

Systemic Retinoid Therapy: A Status Report on Optimal Use and Safety of Long-Term Therapy

Alpesh Desai, DO[a,b,*], Francisca Kartono, BS[b],
James Q. Del Rosso, DO, FAOCD[c]

[a]Heights Dermatology and Aesthetic Center, 2120 Ashland Street, Houston, TX 77008, USA
[b]Western University of Health Sciences, 309 E. Second Street, Pomona, CA 91766, USA
[c]Valley Hospital Medical Center, 620 Shadow Lane, Las Vegas, NY 89106, USA

Retinoids are analogs of vitamin A, whose biological significance was first recognized about 100 years ago [1]. Vitamin A cannot be synthesized in vivo by the human body, and must therefore be obtained exogenously through diet. The important role of vitamin A in epithelial differentiation was observed in the characteristic findings of vitamin A deficiency in humans and animals [2]. Lack of vitamin A induces hyperkeratosis of the skin and squamous metaplasia of mucous membranes, which can be reversed with vitamin A replacement [3]. In 1930, vitamin A was applied therapeutically for treatment of phrynoderma, a characteristic hyperkeratosis with excessive follicular keratinization [4]; however, this effort was complicated by severe hypervitaminosis A syndrome. Unacceptable side effects included skin and mucous membrane changes and bone, liver, and neurologic complications. The low therapeutic index of oral vitamin A and vitamin A acid led to the development of synthetic retinoids.

Today 3 generations of retinoids have been developed. In 1968, investigators began to alter the vitamin A molecule at the polar end group, the polyene side chain, or the cyclic end group of vitamin A. The search for less toxic retinoid derivatives led to the first generation of retinoic acids (RA), which include tretinoin (all-trans-RA), isotretinoin (13-cis-RA), and alitretinoin (9-cis-RA). However, systemic toxicity was not significantly improved over oral vitamin A. In the 1970s, isotretinoin was confirmed to be highly effective against nodulocystic acne and gained approval from the Food and Drug Administration (FDA) in 1982 for the treatment of resistant nodular acne [5].

The second generation of retinoids is composed of aromatic retinoids, by replacing the cyclic end group of vitamin A with various ring systems. In 1986, etretinate was released in the United States for treatment of psoriasis, and by 1998, etretinate was largely replaced by its first metabolite, acitretin. Acitretin seemed to have better pharmacological properties (lower lipid binding, faster elimination). Both aromatic retinoids are highly effective in treating psoriasis and keratinizing skin disorders.

The third generation of retinoic acids includes tazarotene and adapalene, which have been approved by the FDA for topical treatment of psoriasis and acne. Oral tazarotene has been investigated in phase III clinical trials for treatment of psoriasis in adults but has not received FDA approval. Bexarotene is also a third generation retinoic acid, approved for the treatment of cutaneous T-cell lymphoma on adults.

Retinoic acid bioavailability has also been shown to increase with the imidazole derivative liarozole, an inhibitor of cytochrome p-450. Clinical studies showed an effective dose of 75 to 150 mg twice daily in treatment of chronic plaque-type psoriasis [6]. Available oral retinoids in the United States are shown in Table 1 [7–10].

---

* Corresponding author. Heights Dermatology and Aesthetic Center, 2120 Ashland Street, Houston, TX 77008.

E-mail address: drdesai100159@pol.net (A. Desai).

Table 1
Acitretin studies and outcomes on reduction of skin cancer in organ transplant recipients

Retinoid studied	Details	Duration	Conclusion	Reference
Acitretin	N = 1, 0.5 mg/kg/d	15 mo	No new dysplactic lesions	Vandeghinste et al [7]
	N = 38, 30 mg/d	6 mo	Reduction in skin cancer statistically significant	Bouwes-Bavnick et al [8]
	N = 16, 0.3 mg/kg/d	5 y	Reduction in skin cancer statistically significant	McKenna et al [43]
	N = 5, 10–25 mg/d	10–24 mo	Decrease in new tumors compared with pretreatment	McNamara et al [9]
	N = 23, 25 mg/d	2 y	Average 42% increase in skin cancer during drug-free period compared with acitretin period	George et al [10]
	N = 26, 0.2 and 0.4 mg/kg/d	1 y	Decrease in actinic keratoses, no statistical decrease in skin cancer	De Sevaux et al [44]

Pharmacology

General pharmacologic characteristics

Biological effects of retinoids are communicated through cytoplasmic retinoid-binding proteins and nuclear retinoid receptors to activate and regulate gene transcription. There are two classes of nuclear retinoid receptors: the retinoic acid receptor (RAR) and retinoid X receptor (RXR). Each subtype, RAR and RXR receptors, are composed of three different subtypes (α, β, γ) [11]. Additionally, nuclear retinoid receptors exist as dimers, and RARs are known to form heterodimers with RXRs [12]. Both retinoid receptors belong to a large family of receptors consisting of glucocorticosteroid, thyroid hormone, and vitamin D3 receptors, all of which are DNA-binding proteins and function as trans-acting transcription modulating factors [13]. RXR concentration is fivefold higher that RAR concentration in the skin. RXRα/RARγ dimers are postulated as the main regulating complex of retinoid-sensible target genes in adult human skin [14,15].

Mechanism of action

Retinoids modulate and induce the expression of epidermal growth factors. They promote cell differentiation in normal epidermis, but they also act toward normalization of growth in hyperproliferative epithelia. Stimulation of keratinocyte proliferation is expressed by induction of cyclic adenosine monophosphate (cAMP), epidermal growth factor (EGF) receptor binding, protein kinase C, and transforming growth factor alpha (TGF-α). Down-regulation of cell growth on the other hand is regulated by inhibition of epidermal growth factor binding to its receptors, mediated by TGF-β_2. Retinoids are also known to alter terminal differentiation of cells toward a nonkeratinizing, metaplastic, and mucosa-like epithelium [16]. There is a reduction in tonofilaments, a decrease in corneocyte cohesiveness, impairment of permeability barrier function, and an increase in transepidermal water loss, which manifests in the keratolytic effects of retinoids in hyperkeratotic disorders.

Retinoids also exert modifying effects on sebaceous gland activity and epidermal lipids. Isotretinoin has been shown to be effective in reducing sebaceous gland size up to 90% by suppressing the proliferation of basal sebocytes and sebum production in vivo [17]. In vitro studies have confirmed the pronounced and direct inhibitory effect of isotretinoin on the proliferation and lipid synthesis of human sebocytes by controlling their differentiation and antigen expression [18].

Retinoids also exhibit immunomodulatory and anti-inflammatory properties. They are thought to stimulate humoral and cellular immunity by increasing peripheral blood T-cell activity, and enhancing the cytotoxic activity of natural killer cells [19]. It has been demonstrated that acitretin inhibits the migration of polymorphonuclear (PMN) cells by inhibiting their release of reactive oxygen species [20]. In addition, acitretin also decreases the ability of antigen presentation of epidermal cells and decreases the proliferation of phytohemagglutinin-stimulated lymphocytes [21].

Pharmacokinetics

The bioavailability of oral isotretinoin is approximately 25%, and can be increased up to twofold by intake with food [17]. After 30 minutes, the drug is detectable in blood and maximal concentrations are obtained 1 to 4 hours after oral intake.

Etretinate has a bioavailability of 40%, with large interindividual variation because its enteric absorption is enhanced by fat-rich foods. The half-life of isotretinoin ranges from 10 to 20 hours, whereas that of its metabolites ranges from 11 to 50 hours. The half-life of etretinate ranges from 80 to 175 days after multiple doses. The etretinate plasma concentration after a wash-out period of more than 2 years is extremely low and unlikely to be therapeutic; however, it remains potentially teratogenic [22]. Overweight patients tend to have slower elimination rates of etretinate, thereby maintaining higher etretinate serum concentrations because of prolonged clearance [23]. This is likely attributable to sequestration in body fat stores followed by prolonged delayed redistribution into the systemic circulation.

Use of oral retinoids

Acne

Isotretinoin is currently available as the most effective retinoid against acne vulgaris. Isotretinoin is indicated for nodular acne that is refractory to conventional therapy, including systemic antibiotics and topical regimens. Oral isotretinoin therapy is usually prescribed over an average duration of 20 weeks, depending on the daily dosage used (see below).

Isotretinoin has been shown to be superior to erythromycin and to combination of oral tetracycline and topical retinoic acid [24,25]. Most patients experience complete or dramatic prolonged clearance of acne vulgaris lasting for several years after discontinuation of treatment. Relapses can occur at any time after discontinuation, with a reported rate approximately of 21% [26,27]. Oral isotretinoin remains a highly effective drug for acne treatment. Although there is potential for significant side effects, most patients do not experience major adverse events when isotretinoin is properly prescribed and use is appropriately monitored.

Acute flares of acne may occur in some patients after initiation of isotretinoin treatment. Such flares can be reduced by initiating therapy with a starting dose of 0.5 mg/kg/day as opposed to 1 mg/kg/day, and with the concomitant use of an oral antibiotic during the first 4 weeks of treatment [28]. Tetracyclines are not recommended in combination with oral isotretinoin because of an alleged increased risk of pseudotumor cerebri, although confirmatory data supporting this premise is lacking. Regardless of the exact dosing regimen ranging from 0.5 to 1 mg/kg daily, a cumulative dose of 120 mg/kg is recommended to reduce the chance of relapse after isotretinoin therapy [28].

Psoriasis

Etretinate and its metabolite acitretin have been FDA-approved for the treatment of psoriasis in adults, with the most rapid and consistent response seen with monotherapy in the pustular and erythrodermic types. Acitretin has mainly replaced etretinate in the treatment of psoriasis and has shown activity when used in combination, rotational, and sequential therapy regimens with other therapies [29]. In psoriasis patients treated with extensive exposure to psoralen ultraviolet A (PUVA), acitretin has been shown to reduce the number of treatments needed and the total amount of UV exposure required to achieve beneficial results and also decreases the occurrence of squamous cell carcinomas. The combination of acitretin or etretinate with PUVA (RePUVA) as psoriasis therapy has been shown to yield more rapid clearance of severe plaque psoriasis, with decreased cumulative dose of both medications when compared with either modality as a monotherapy [30]. Similar results have been obtained using acitretin and ultraviolet B (ReUVB) [31,32]. Overall toxicity profile is better with ReUVB, however RePUVA has shown to be more effective in recalcitrant psoriasis [33].

Currently acitretin is the only oral retinoid currently approved for psoriasis, and is effective as monotherapy in pustular, erythrodermic, and plaque psoriasis; the efficacy of acitretin is maintained with repeated courses of use [34]. It is active alone and in combination with phototherapy (UVB, PUVA, narrowband UVB), topical agents, and systemic methotrexate and cyclosporine. It is notable that acitretin is currently the only existing FDA-approved systemic psoriasis therapy that is not an immunosuppressant [13]. In psoriasis patients who have concomitant chronic infections and thus are immunosuppressed, acitretin becomes a safer treatment option not offered by the current advent of biological agents.

A recent study by Pearce and colleagues [35] evaluated the reduction in acitretin-associated adverse effects with low dose treatment (25 mg/day) in psoriasis patients as compared with adverse effect rates associated with higher doses ($\geq$ 50 mg/day). The findings concluded that with a 25 mg/day treatment dose, efficacy was maintained with a significant reduction in side effects when compared with 50 mg/day or greater. Low dose acitretin therapy is less likely to result in discontinuation of treatment because of adverse events, such as alopecia or increase in serum triglyceride levels.

Disorders of keratinization

First and second generation retinoids are also effective in other disorders of keratinization besides psoriasis, since their action in promoting keratinocytic differentiation is not specific for psoriasis [17].

Oral retinoids have been shown to normalize hyperkeratotic and dyskeratotic conditions, including severe genetic disorders of keratinization. Treatment of young patients specifically with genodermatoses has been shown to improve their quality of life, enhance social and psychologic development, and also improve height and weight gain while on oral retinoids [36]. A 90% to 100% improvement has been reported with 1 to 2 mg/kg/d of etretinate in children with lamellar ichtyoses, keratosis follicularis (Darier's disease), pityiasis rubra pilaris, symmetric progressive keratoderma, and palmoplantar keratoderma [37]. In epidermolytic hyperkeratosis, a remission rate of 70% to 80% was observed [37]. There have also been case reports of infants with harlequin ichtyosis who have survived on etretinate or acitretin. The most common reported side effects were mucocutaneous dryness and minor liver and triglyceride laboratory abnormalities, with no reported irreversible side effects [38].

Skin cancer

Oral retinoids have been used to decrease the rate and level of development of cutaneous malignancies and genodermatoses, such as xeroderma pigmentosum, nevoid basal cell carcinoma syndrome, and epidermoplasia verruciformis [39]; however, a rebound effect has been reported after discontinuation of the retinoid therapy [40]. Older reports included patients treated with high doses, such as 75 mg or more daily of acitretin, which was associated with a high potential for intolerability because of side effects. Many patients with psoriasis or disorders of keratinization, those with genetic susceptibility to multiple skin cancers such as SCCs, and in organ transplant recipients or phototherapy patients who exhibit frequent development of SCCs, low dose acitretin (25 mg daily) is often effective in controlling their disease. Low dose acitretin is associated with a much lower frequency of side effects and is well tolerated by most patients, even with chronic use [35]. Based on therapeutic response, some patients may require a progressive escalation of their acitretin dose to 35 mg to 50 mg daily.

Organ transplant patients who are immunosuppressed are at higher risk of developing nonmelanoma skin cancers, of which squamous cell skin cancer is the most common [41]. The squamous cell carcinomas in this subset of patients tend to be multiple, with frequent recurrence and have a more aggressive course. Clinical studies have agreed on the beneficial effect of acitretin in reducing premalignant keratoses, and most case reports and quasi-controlled case series have supported the statistically significant effect of acitretin in reducing SCC. No controlled randomized trials currently exist to quantify the therapeutic effect and minimal effective dosing; however, a dosage range of 25 to 50 mg daily is often efficacious [42]. Based on the adverse effects such as headaches, rash, cheleitis, elevation in lipid profile, and osteoporosis, initiation of therapy should begin at the lowest dose and advance to an effective maintenance dose according to the patient's clinical response and side-effect profile. Despite poor tolerability as the major limitation to the use of systemic retinoids in transplant patients, especially with higher doses, discontinuation of treatment because of adverse effects has only been seen in a minimal population. The theoretical increased chance of allograft rejection because of the immunopotentiating effects of retinoid therapy has not been substantiated [43,44].

The reported optimal dosing of acitretin for chemoprevention in transplant patients has ranged from as low as 0.18 mg/kg/day to 0.5 mg/kg/day, or in daily doses of 10 mg per day to 50 mg per day alternating with 25 mg daily [45]. A rebound effect, characterized by a return to the pretreatment frequency of SCC development, should be expected with discontinuation of acitretin treatment, making continuous long-term therapy necessary in these patients to sustain suppression of new tumor formation. A recent retrospective study on the effects of acitretin (0.2 to 0.4 mg/kg/d) in transplant patients after 1 to 16 years of treatment reported a statistically significant reduction in SCCs for the first 3 years, and further reduction in subsequent years that was not statistically significant [46]. The study did not find a major effect of age, duration of transplantation, and duration of first SCC until initiation of retinoid therapy on their efficacy [46].

Interestingly, a study by De Sevaux and colleagues [44] noted no improvement in the reduction of SCCs in renal transplant patients despite reducing the number of actinic keratoses; however, no control group was used in this study. The few number of available controlled studies have supported that acitretin has marked therapeutic potential as an effective chemoprophylactic agent in organ transplant recipients with appropriate selection of patients and careful use of dosage regimens to decrease the risk of side effects.

Guidelines by the International Transplant Skin Cancer Collaborative and European Skin Care in Organ Transplant Patients Network recommend systemic retinoid therapy as chemoprophylaxis in transplant patients to reduce the occurrence of squamous cell carcinoma in organ transplant patients [47]. A decrease in the number of squamous cell carcinoma allows this subset of patients to benefit from an improved quality of life and decreased morbidity.

Acitretin has also been useful in the prevention of squamous cell carcinomas caused by PUVA therapy and in the treatment of arsenical keratoses and Bowen's disease [48,49]. The efficacy of systemic retinoids in chemoprevention of skin cancers requires long-term therapy. Multiple new tumors have been observed upon discontinuation of a retinoid regimen, which diminish upon reintroduction of the drug [50]. Benefits and long-term side effects of acitretin as a chemopreventive agent warrant further investigation.

Side effects of oral retinoids

Side effects of oral retinoids have a clinical spectrum similar to chronic hypervitaminosis A syndrome, affecting numerous organ systems. The concern regarding safety of long-term therapy has developed because patients with genodermatoses may require lifelong therapy. In separating short-term from long-term side effects, "long-term" side effects has been defined as those that appear after more than 1 year of therapy, either during continuous or intermittent treatment over several years. The main organ systems at risk from long-term side effects of oral retinoid therapy generally include the liver and musculoskeletal and cardiovascular systems [51,52]. Other common side effects of systemic retinoids are briefly reviewed.

Hepatotoxicity

Oral retinoids may be hepatotoxic with two types identified: pseudoallergic (idiosyncratic) hepatitis or low-grade (pharmacologic) hepatotoxicity [51]. Prospective biopsy studies of patients treated with etretinate have not indicated clear-cut progression of both types of hepatotoxicity to cirrhosis.

Elevated transaminases have been reported to occur in approximately 15% of patients on oral retinoid therapy [45]. Elevated liver enzyme levels are generally mild and reversible within 2 to 4 weeks despite continued retinoid therapy [3].

It has been recommended that acitretin and methotrexate not be used concurrently because of increased potential for hepatotoxicity.

Musculoskeletal

Diffuse skeletal hyperostosis (DISH syndrome), remodeling of long bones, decalcification, progressive calcification of ligaments and tendon insertions, periosteal thickening, premature epiphyseal closure, and possible osteoporosis have been reported. DISH syndrome manifestations include anterior spinal ligament calcification, osteophytes, and bony bridges without narrowing of the disk space; however, the aforementioned ostoses have been shown to be common in individuals in the general population who have never been treated with systemic retinoids [53].

Myalgias, arthralgias, and back pain have been reported in patients taking oral retinoids [54]. Elevated creatinine phosphokinase (CPK) as a benign phenomenon and associated with rhabdomyolysis were also reported in several patients on isotretinoin [55,56].

The most alarming bone change is premature epiphyseal closure in children treated with isotretinoin. This irreversible side effect has been reported after high-dose therapy for disorders of keratinization and appears to take at least 1 year to develop. Retinoid therapy in children and adolescents should be distinguished between short-term and long-term therapy. Studies have shown that a 20-week course of isotretinoin for nodulocystic acne is generally well tolerated and safe [3]. Bony side effects with short-term therapy is rare. On the other hand, long-term therapy with etretinate and acitretin for disorders of keratinization may result in skeletal toxicities, especially in children, and should be used with caution.

Cardiovascular

Cardiovascular side effects of retinoids are related to the changes seen in lipid metabolism with the use of systemic retinoids. Markedly elevated levels of triglycerides and mild elevation of HDL and total cholesterol have been reported with the use of retinoids. It has been reported that isotretinoin-induced elevations in triglycerides were dose-dependent and reversible within 8 weeks after the cessation of the drug [57].

The hyperlipidemic potential of isotretinoin appears to be somewhat higher than for etretinate or acitretin, but because isotretinoin is given in young persons and for less than 1 year, the problems with long-term safety may be less evident than for the aromatic retinoids, which are predominantly used in older patients.

Mucocutaneous

Toxicities most commonly observed include cheilitis and dryness of the nasal mucosa, which can sometimes lead to epistaxis. Cheilitis is the most common manifestation, especially with isotretinoin, and it has been stated that absence of cheilitis in a patient treated with isotretinoin for acne should raise marked suspicion of noncompliance with treatment [58]. Periungual granulation tissue formation at sites of paronychia has also been reported [59]. Xeroderma, arthralgia, dry eye syndrome, and eczema exacerbation have been considered as long-term side effects of isotretinoin [60]. Diffuse hair thinning, brittle nails, palmar and plantar desquamation, and increased skin fragility have also been associated [61]. Mucocutaneous toxicities are generally dose-dependent and reversible on discontinuation of therapy.

Teratogenicity

All systemic retinoids are assigned a pregnancy category X by the FDA. Birth defects induced by retinoids or retinoic acid embryopathy include central nervous system abnormalities, external ear abnormalities, cardiovascular abnormalities, facial dysmorphia, eye abnormalities, thymus gland abnormalities, and bone abnormalities.

To minimize the number of isotretinoin-exposed pregnancies, the FDA's Drug Safety and Risk Management Advisory Committee and Dermatologic and Ophthalmic Drugs Advisory Committee implemented a mandatory program that requires registration in iPLEDGE by licensed prescribers and patients who agree to accept specific responsibilities before receiving authorization to prescribe or use the drug [62]. Wholesalers and pharmacies must also comply with the manufacturers' program requirements to distribute and dispense the product.

As with etretinate, use of acitretin is not recommended in females of childbearing potential; however, in cases of mitigating circumstances warranting treatment based on risk versus benefit assessment, such female patients treated with acitretin must undergo baseline evaluation and testing to ensure that they are not pregnant before starting therapy. Also, they must use two effective forms of contraception before, during, and for up to 3 years after completion of acitretin treatment. In male patients, it has not been elucidated whether acitretin in seminal fluid would pose a risk to the developing fetus. There is currently no FDA requirement for male patients taking acitretin.

Pseudotumor cerebri

Benign intracranial hypertension, or pseudotumor cerebri, has been linked to the use of systemic retinoids. Symptoms include papilledema, severe headaches, nausea and vomiting, and visual disturbances. Concomitant intake of tetracycline or its derivatives has been stated to promote the risk of pseudotumor cerebri and should be avoided according to product labeling, although data are limited. Tetracycline antibiotics have been suggested to decrease cerebrospinal fluid reabsorption by affecting cAMP at the arachnoid villi [63]. The precise incidence of this side effect remains unclear. The paucity of case reports has not proven a certain causal relationship [57]; however, symptoms strongly suggestive of papilledema and/or a positive ophthalmologic exam for papilledema warrant discontinuation of retinoid use.

Psychiatric effects

To date, there has been no convincing scientific publication establishing an association between depression and oral retinoids. The risk of depression has resulted in the addition of a precaution on the acitretin package insert since April 2003 [64]. Case reports and anecdotal sources have associated isotretinoin therapy and depression [65]. In a pilot study, functional brain imaging changes have been shown to occur in patients undergoing isotretinoin therapy, although the significance of these data is unclear [66]. However, there is still a lack of convincing evidence base for acitretin-associated depression and self-injurious behavior [67].

Dosage initiation and monitoring

Isotretinoin

Isotretinoin therapy for refractory nodulocystic acne is best initiated at a dose of 0.5 mg/kg daily. The rapidity of response to treatment varies from patient to patient. Some patients demonstrate progressive improvement that is visibly evident as early as 4 to 6 weeks. Others respond more slowly. After a few months, the dose may be increased to 1 mg/kg daily in slower responders.

In some cases, an initial flare may occur soon after starting oral isotretinoin treatment. When severe, this initial exacerbation may be temporized by use of short-course oral corticosteroid therapy and should not trigger an increase in isotretinoin dosage.

Baseline liver enzyme testing, lipid profile, and pregnancy testing (in females) is recommended and should be repeated monthly during the course of therapy.

The duration of isotretinoin therapy averages approximately 20 weeks in many patients. The therapeutic end point is generally reached once a total cumulative dose for a given course of oral isotretinoin therapy reaches 120 to 150 mg/kg.

All patients using oral isotretinoin therapy must comply with the details mandated by the iPLEDGE program. Special requirements apply to females of childbearing potential, which relate to adequate contraception before, during, and for 1 month after cessation of therapy; pregnancy testing and reporting requirements are also mandated by the program.

Acitretin

Many strategies can be used to prevent or reduce the long-term side effects of oral acitretin therapy. Depending on the disease state, combination or intermittent therapy allows for minimal dosing. Use of low-dose acitretin therapy has been shown to markedly reduce side effects without loss of efficacy. Laboratory and physical findings should be monitored regularly.

Initial clinical monitoring should require examination every 4 weeks to assess and manage potential mucocutaneous and other side effects, ensure compliance, and evaluate monitored laboratory parameters. In general, liver enzyme and blood lipids should be measured every 4 to 8 weeks, and adjusted thereafter based on clinical judgment correlated with the individual patient. Retinoid dosing should be adjusted or interrupted when significant elevations in laboratory indices occur. Appropriate selection of patients and diet schedules can be used as precautions to reduce the risk of hyperlipidemia. Particularly with young patients on long-term retinoid therapy, regular radiological examination of the skeletal system may be necessary.

The use of acitretin is best avoided in females of childbearing potential; however, as stated earlier, in cases deemed to warrant treatment, female patients treated with acitretin who are capable of becoming pregnant must undergo baseline evaluation and testing to ensure that they are not pregnant before starting therapy. Also, they must use two effective forms of contraception before, during, and for up to 3 years after completion of acitretin treatment.

Summary

Systemic retinoids are an important component of the dermatology treatment armamentarium offering unique therapeutic properties, and are widely used to treat a large spectrum of skin disorders. Rational selection of candidates for treatment, knowledge regarding appropriate and optimal use, awareness of common and uncommon potential adverse reactions, and proper use of clinical and laboratory monitoring can result in effective and safe treatment of several severe skin disorders that impact poorly on the overall health and quality of life of affected patients.

References

[1] Wolbach S, Howe P. Tissue changes following deprivation of fat-soluble A-vitamin. J Exp Med 1925; 42:753–78.

[2] Giudice G, Fuchs E. Vitamin A-mediated regulation of keratinocyte differentiation. Methods Enzymol 1990;190:18–29.

[3] Brecher A, Orlow S. Oral retinoid therapy for dermatologic conditions in children and adolescents. J Am Acad Dermatol 2003;49:171–82.

[4] Gollnick H, Dummler U. Retinoids. Clin Dermatol 1997;15:799–810.

[5] Peck G, Yoder F, Strauss J, et al. Prolonged remissions of cystic and conglobata acne with 13-*cis*-retinoic acid. N Engl J Med 1979;300:329–33.

[6] Dockx P, Decree J, Degreef H. Inhibition of the metabolism of endogenous retinoic acid as treatment for severe psoriasis: an open study with oral liarozole. Br J Dermatol 1995;133:426–32.

[7] Vandeghinste N, De Bersaques J, Geerts M, et al. Acitretin as cancer chemoprophylaxis in a renal transplant recipient. Dermatology 1992;185:307–8.

[8] Bavinck JN, Tieben LM, Van der Woude FJ, et al. Prevention of skin cancer and reduction of keratotic skin lesions during acitretin therapy in renal transplant recipients: a double-blind placebo controlled study. J Clin Oncol 1995;13:1933–1938.

[9] McNamara I, Muir J, Galbraith A. Acitretin for prophylaxis of cutaneous malignancies after cardiac transplantation. J Heart Lung Transplant 2002;21: 1201–5.

[10] George R, Weightman W, Russ GR, et al. Acitretin for chemoprevention of non-melanoma skin cancers in renal transplant recipients. Australas J Dermatol 2002;43:269–73.

[11] Chambon P. The retinoid signaling pathway: molecular and genetic analysis. Semin Cell Biol 1994;5: 115–25.

[12] Saurat K. Retinoids and psoriasis: novel issues in retinoid pharmacology and implications for psoriasis treatment. J Am Acad Dermatol 1999;41:S2–6.

[13] Lee C, Koo J. A review of acitretin, a systemic retinoid for the treatment of psoriasis. Expert Opin Pharmacother 2005;6(10):1725–34.

[14] Fisher G, Talwar H, Xiao J, et al. Immunological identification and functional quantitation of retinoic acid and retinoid X receptor protein in human skin. J Biol Chem 1994;269:20629–35.

[15] Xiao J, Durand B, Chambon P, et al. Endogenous retinoic acid receptor (RAR)-retinoid X receptor (RXR) heterodimers are the major functional forms in adult human keratinocytes. J Biol Chem 1995;270: 2001–11.

[16] Griffiths C, Dabelsteen E, Voorhees J. Topical retinoic acid changes the epidermal cell surface glycosylation pattern towards that of a mucosal epithelium. Br J Dermatol 1996;134:431–6.

[17] Orfanos C, Zouboulis C, Almond-Roesler B, et al. Current use and future potential role of retinoids in dermatology. Drugs 1997;53(3):358–88.

[18] Zouboulis C, Korge B, Akamatsu H, et al. Effects of 13-*cis*-retinoic acid, all-trans-retinoic acid, and acitretin on the proliferation, lipid synthesis and keratin expression of cultured human sebocytes *in vitro*. J Invest Dermatol 1991;96:792–7.

[19] Kempf W, Kettelhack N, Duvic M, et al. Topical and systemic retinoid therapy for cutaneous T-cell lymphoma. Hematol Oncol Clin North Am 2003; 17:1405–19.

[20] Struy H, Bohne M, Morenz J, et al. Effects of retinoids on human neutrophil derived free radicals. Eur J Haematol 1996;59(Suppl 57):52.

[21] Dupuy P, Bagot M, Heslan M, et al. Synthetic retinoids inhibit the antigen presenting properties of epidermal cells in vitro. J Invest Dermatol 1989; 93:455–9.

[22] Chalmers R. Retinoid therapy—a real hazard for the developing embryo. Br J Obstet Gynaecol 1992;99: 276–8.

[23] DiGiovanna J, Zech L, Ruddel M, et al. Etretinate. Persistent serum levels after long-term therapy. Arch Dermatol 1989;125:246–51.

[24] Jones D. A comparison of 13-cis-retinoic acid and erythromycin treatment in severe acne. Br J Dermatol 1983;109(Suppl 24):27–8.

[25] Langner A, Wolska H, Fraczykowska M, et al. 13-cis-retinoic acid and tetracycline versus 13-cis-retinoic acid alone in the treatment of nodulocystic acne. Dermatologica 1985;170(4):185–8.

[26] Wessels F, Anderson AN, Kropman K. The cost-effectiveness of isotretinoin in the treatment of acne. Part I. A meta-analysis of effectiveness literature. S Afr Med J 1999;89(7 Pt 2):780–4.

[27] Chivot M, Midoun H. Isotretinoin and acne—a study of relapses. Dermatologica 1990;180(4):240–3.

[28] Charakida A, Mouser PE, Chu AC. Safety and side effects of the acne drug, oral isotretinoin. Expert Opin Drug Saf 2004;3(2):119–29.

[29] Lebwohl M, Kathryn M. New roles for systemic retinoids. J Drugs Dermatol 2006;5(5):406–9.

[30] Saurat J, Geiger J, Amblard P, et al. Randomized double-blind multi-center study comparing acitretin-PUVA, etretinate-PUVA, and placebo-PUVA in the treatment of severe psoriasis. Dermatologica 1988;177:218–24.

[31] Iest J, Boer J. Combined treatment of psoriasis with acitretin alone and UVB phototherapy compared with acitretin alone and UVB alone. Br J Dermatol 1989;120:665–70.

[32] Ruzicka T, Sommerburg C, Braun-Falco O, et al. Efficiency of acitretin in combination with UV-B in the treatment of severe psoriasis. Arch Dermatol 1990;126:482–6.

[33] Green C, Lakshmipathi T, Johnson B, et al. A comparison of the efficacy and relapse rates of narrowband UVB (TL-01) monotherapy vs. etretinate (re-TL-01) vs. etretinate-PUVA (re-PUVA) in the treatment of psoriasis patients. Br J Dermatol 1992;127:5–9.

[34] Stebbins W, Lebwohl M. Biologics in combination with nonbiologics: efficacy and safety. Dermatol Ther 2004;17:432–40.

[35] Pearce D, Klinger S, Ziel K, et al. Low-dose acitretin is associated with fewer adverse events than high-dose acitretin in the treatment of psoriasis. Arch Dermatol 2006;142:1000–4.

[36] Ruiz-Maldonado R, Tamayo L. Retinoids in disorders of keratinization: their use in children. Dermatologica 1987;175:123–32.

[37] Tamayo L, Ruiz-Maldonado R, et al. Long-term follow-up of 30 children under oral retinoid Ro 10-9359. In: Orfanos CE, Braun-Falco O, Farber EM, editors. Retinoids: advances in basic research and therapy. Berlin: Springer-Verlag; 1981. p. 287–94.

[38] Blanchet-Bardon C, Nazarro V, Rognin C, et al. Acitretin in the treatment of severe disorders of keratinization. J Am Acad Dermatol 1991;24:982–6.

[39] Bollag W, Holdener E. Retinoids in cancer prevention and therapy. Ann Oncol 1992;3(7):513–26.

[40] Peck G. Long-term retinoid therapy is needed for maintenance of cancer chemopreventive effect. Dermatologica 1987;175(Suppl 1):138–44.

[41] Euvrard S, Kanitakis J, Claudy A. Skin cancers after organ transplantation. N Engl J Med 2003;348:1681–91.

[42] Chen K, Craig J, Shumack S. Oral retinoids for the prevention of skin cancers in solid organ transplant recipients: a systematic review of randomized controlled trials. Br J Dermatol 2005;152:518–23.

[43] Mc Kenna D, Murphy G. Skin cancer chemprophylaxis in renal transplant recipients: 5 years of experience using low-dose acitretin. Br J Dermatol 1999;140:656–60.

[44] De Sevaux R, Smit J, De Jong E, et al. Acitretin treatment of premalignant and malignant skin disorders in renal transplant recipients: clinical effects of a randomized trial comparing two doses of acitretin. J Am Acad Dermatol 2003;49:407–12.

[45] Kovach B, Sams H, Stasko T. Systemic strategies for chemoprevention of skin cancers in transplant recipients. Clin Transplant 2005;19(6):726–34.

[46] Harwood C, Leedham-Green M, Leigh I, et al. Low-dose retinoids in the prevention of cutaneous squamous cell carcinomas in organ transplant recipients. Arch Dermatol 2005;141:456–64.

[47] Stasko T, Brown M, Carucci J, et al. Guidelines for the management of squamous cell carcinoma in organ transplant recipients. Dermatol Surg 2004;30:642–50.

[48] Van de Kerkhof P, de Rooij MJ. Multiple squamous cell carcinomas in a psoriatic patient following high-dose photochemotherapy and cyclosporine treatment: response to long-term acitretin maintenance. Br J Dermatol 1997;136:275–8.

[49] Yerebakan O, Ermis O, Yilmaz E, et al. Treatment of arsenical keratosis and Bowen's disease with acitretin. Int J Dermatol 2002;41(2):84–7.

[50] Lebwohl M, Tannis C, Carrasco D. Acitretin suppression of squamous cell carcinoma: a case report and literature review. J Dermatol Treat 2003;14(Suppl 2):3–6.

[51] Vahlquist A. Long-term safety of retinoid therapy. J Am Acad Dermatol 1992;27:S29–33.

[52] Ellis C, Krach K. Uses and complications of isotretinoin therapy. J Am Acad Dermatol 2001;45(Suppl):S150–7.

[53] Jones M, Pais M, Omiya B. Bony overgrowths and abnormal calcifications about the spine. Radiol Clin North Am 1988;26:1213–34.

[54] Peck G, DiGiovanna J, et al. The retinoids. In: Freedberg I, Eisen A, editors. Dermatology in general medicine. New York: McGraw-Hill; 1999. p. 2810–20.

[55] Heudes A, Laroche L. Muscular damage during isotretinoin treatment. Ann Dermatol Venereol 1998;125:94–7.

[56] Landau M, Mesterman R, Ophir J, et al. Clinical significance of markedly elevated creatinine kinase levels in patients with acne on isotretinoin. Acta Derm Venereol 2001;81:350–2.

[57] US Food and Drug Administration. Isotretinoin (marketed as Accutane) capsule information. October 2006. Available at: http://www.fda.gov/cder/drug/infopage/accutane/default.htm. Accessed June 11, 2006.

[58] Exner J, Dahod S, Pochi P. Pyogenic granuloma-like acne lesions during isotretinoin therapy. Arch Dermatol 1983;119:808–11.

[59] Bigby M, Stern R. Adverse reactions to isotretinoin: a report from the adverse drug reaction reporting system. J Am Acad Dermatol 1988;18:543–52.

[60] Goulden V, Laytom A, Cunliffe W. Long-term safety of isotretinoin as a treatment for acne vulgaris. Br J Dermatol 1994;131:360–3.

[61] Nguyen E, Wolverton S. Systemic retinoids. In: Wolverton S, Wilkin J, editors. Systemic drugs for skin diseases. Philadelphia: WB Saunders; 2000. p. 269–310.

[62] Weinberg J. iPLEDGE allegiance. Cutis 2005;76(6):356.

[63] Stuart B, Litt I. Tetracycline-associated intracranial hypertension in an adolescent: a complication of systemic acne therapy. J Pediatr 1978;92:679–80.

[64] Soriatane, inventor. Connetics Corporation, assignee [Package insert]. Palo Alto (CA); 2003.

[65] Bleiker T, Bourke J, Graham-Brown R, et al. Etretinate may work where acitretin fails. Br J Dermatol 1997;136(3):368–70.

[66] Bremner J, Fani N, Ashraf A, et al. Functional brain imaging alterations in acne patients treated with isotretinoin. Am J Psychiatry 2005;162(5):983–91.

[67] Starling J III, Koo J. Evidence based or theoretical concern? Pseudotumor cerebri and depression as acitretin side effects. J Drugs Dermatol 2005;4(6):690–6.

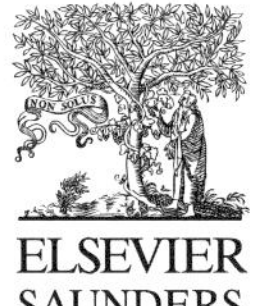

DERMATOLOGIC
CLINICS

Dermatol Clin 25 (2007) 195–205

Suggested Guidelines for Patient Monitoring: Hepatic and Hematologic Toxicity Attributable to Systemic Dermatologic Drugs

Stephen E. Wolverton, MD[a],*, Kathleen Remlinger, MD[b]

[a]Indiana University Medical Center, Department of Dermatology, 550 N. University Boulevard, Suite 3240, Indianapolis, IN 46202, USA
[b]Rush-Presbyterian-St. Luke's Medical Center, 1653 W. Congress Parkway, Chicago, IL 60612, USA

Hepatic and hematologic toxicity are among the most fearful adverse effects that occasionally occur as a result of systemic drugs in the dermatologist's therapeutic armamentarium. Drugs of greatest interest concerning hepatic toxicity include methotrexate, azathioprine, dapsone, and acitretin. Somewhat overlapping are drugs that have important hematologic toxicities, including methotrexate, azathioprine, dapsone, sulfonamides, cyclophosphamide, and chlorambucil. Laboratory tests commonly used include (1) hepatic monitoring: transaminases (apartate aminotransferase/serum glutamate oxaloacetate transaminase [AST/SGOT] and alanine aminotransferase/serum glutamate pyruvate transaminase [ALT/SGPT]) and ultrasound-guided liver biopsy, and (2) hematologic monitoring: complete blood count (CBC) with differential and platelets along with occasional use of the reticulocyte count. Important principles and specific guidelines for monitoring by drug group are highlighted.

Overview of hepatic toxicity

Incidence and categories

The importance of drug-induced liver disease (drug hepatotoxicity) is illustrated by the following statistics [1,2]: (1) drugs are estimated to be responsible for 10% of cases of hepatitis in adults, (2) drugs are responsible for about 40% to 50% of cases of hepatitis in adults at least 50 years old,

(3) it is estimated that at least 25% of all cases of fulminant hepatitis are attributable to drugs, and (4) liver failure, when it is drug-induced on an idiosyncratic basis, is fatal 75% to 80% of the time [3]. The four major subsets of drug-induced liver disease include (1) hepatocellular toxicity, (2) drug hypersensitivity syndrome, (3) cholestasis, and (4) steatosis progressing to fibrosis.

Mechanisms of drug hepatotoxicity

The most well-accepted hypothesis explaining idiosyncratic drug-induced liver disease has two components [4]. First, there must be the presence of reactive metabolic intermediates, which are electrophilic compounds that rapidly form covalent bonds to various cellular components if not equally rapidly detoxified. Second, there generally must be a defect in the cellular detoxification systems for there to be an adequate presence or persistence of these reactive intermediates to result in significant hepatic pathology.

Two potential outcomes are thought to occur when there are excessive quantities of reactive, electrophilic intermediates [5,6]. First is the potential for direct toxicity to neighboring cells (most notably the hepatocyte) from protein, DNA, and lipid biomembrane alterations resulting from covalent binding to these intermediates. Second, the covalent binding of the reactive intermediates to various proteins leads to the development of new antigens (neoantigens) [7]. These neoantigens can include various CYP isoforms that logically are "in the neighborhood" when the reactive intermediates are created [8,9].

* Corresponding author.
E-mail address: swolvert@iupui.edu (S.E. Wolverton).

Direct drug-induced *toxicity* to the liver merely results from excessive drug levels from very few specific drugs [5,10]. The classic liver toxicity example is an acetaminophen overdose, although pharmacologic doses of acetaminophen in the presence of a CYP 2E1 inducer (chronic excessive ethanol consumption) can produce a similar result. In contrast, the term *idiosyncratic* suggests that only a distinct minority of individuals will experience drug-induced liver disease from selected drugs, and that the reaction will occur independent of drug dose. Under this heading is where the vast majority of hepatotoxicity caused by drugs occurs [11,12].

Risk factors for drug hepatotoxicity

There are a number of factors, aside from genetic predisposition/idiosyncrasy, which help explain why some individuals react to a given medication while the majority of patients do not. A classic example would be the increased probability of methotrexate hepatotoxicity (steatosis → fibrosis) in the setting of one or more of the following potential risk factors: excessive ethanol consumption, obesity, diabetes mellitus, and renal insufficiency [13,14].

Daily dose is probably a factor in systemic retinoid hepatotoxicity [15], whereas cumulative dose is a key determinant of risk for methotrexate-induced liver disease [13,14]. Timing from the onset of drug administration is critical in laboratory surveillance for drugs that can cause the drug hypersensitivity syndrome (DHS), such as azathioprine [16], dapsone [17,18], and minocycline [19,20]. Idiosyncratic reactions to ketoconazole, albeit lacking other components of the DHS, occur in a similar timing most notably between weeks 3 and 12 of drug administration, particularly in the first half of this time interval. Ketoconazole will not be discussed further in this chapter, given the far safer azole and allylamine antifungal agents currently available.

Classification systems

The ideal classification system would be based on clinical and laboratory evidence of liver disease, liver histology, and full awareness of the mechanism behind various patterns of drug-induced liver disease. Laboratory test abnormalities suggesting hepatobiliary obstruction (cholestasis) are distinctly uncommon from systemic drugs used in dermatology. A liver biopsy is routinely indicated only for patients on long-term methotrexate therapy.

Laboratory evidence for both hepatocellular toxicity and DHS patients is similar (Table 1).

Specific approaches to hepatic toxicity monitoring

Background information

Liver "function" tests

The phrase "liver function tests" (LFTs) is clearly a misnomer given that the most commonly used LFT, the transaminases, merely measure hepatocyte integrity and may be elevated by abnormalities in distant organs [21–23]. Tests listed in Table 2 that measure hepatic protein synthesis (international normalized ratio [INR] or albumin levels) do measure one aspect of liver function; however, these tests are still not ideally specific, and are typically abnormal only late in the disease course. For most systemic drugs discussed in this chapter that are commonly prescribed by dermatologists, the combination of serum AST/SGOT

Table 1
Major categories of liver toxicity attributable to drugs

Category	Best diagnostic tests	Dermatologic drugs
Hepatocellular	AST/SGOT ALT/SGPT	Ketoconazole Dapsone Minocycline Azathioprine Acitretin Methotrexate[a]
Hypersensitivity Syndrome	AST/SGOT ALT/SGPT Eosinophil count	Dapsone Minocycline Azathioprine Sulfonamides
Cholestasis	Alkaline phosphatase GGT Bilirubin (conjugated)	Erythromycin estolate TMP-SMX
Steatosis → Fibrosis (macrovesicular)	Liver biopsy Transaminases	Methotrexate Acitretin (rarely)

Abbreviations: GGT, γ-glutamyl transpeptidase; TMP-SMX, trimethoprim-sulfamethoxazole.

[a] Methotrexate will occasionally induce hepatocellular toxicity, although it is generally mild-moderate in severity.

Adapted from Wolverton SE. Hepatotoxicity due to dermatologic drugs. In: Wolverton SE, editor. Comprehensive dermatologic drug therapy. 2nd edition. London: Elsevier; 2007. p. 877–92.

Table 2
Most commonly used "liver function tests"

Test name	Comments/limitations
Tests for hepatocyte integrity	
AST/SGOT	Less specific for the liver than ALT/SGPT
ALT/SGPT	More specific for the liver than AST/SGOT
Tests for hepatobiliary obstruction	
Alkaline phosphatase	Nonspecific for liver (also found in bone); lab can fractionate to increase specificity
Bilirubin	Later finding in setting of hepatobiliary obstruction; hemolysis gives "false positives"
Tests of hepatic protein synthesis	
Albumin	Very late, yet important sign of reduced liver function
Protime/INR	Very late, yet important sign of reduced liver function
Test for "severity" of liver failure	
Ammonia	Very late sign of severe, often end-stage liver disease; marker for encephalopathy
Test for ongoing fibrosis	
P3NP[a]	False positives from other sites of fibrosis (such as psoriatic arthritis)

Abbreviation: P3NP, aminoterminus of type 3 collagen propeptide.

[a] The P3NP test is currently available in many European Union countries, but not yet commercially available in the US.

Adapted from Wolverton SE. Hepatotoxicity due to dermatologic drugs. In: Wolverton SE, editor. Comprehensive dermatologic drug therapy. 2nd edition. London: Elsevier; 2007. p. 877–92.

and ALT/SGPT (the "transaminases") remain the standard of care for laboratory surveillance. In complicated cases in which patients approach or pass the critical level of threefold transaminase elevation or if there are persistent abnormalities in the transaminase values, the clinician is encouraged to seek gastroenterology or hepatology consultation (Table 2).

Differential diagnosis

It is important to consider at least four other possibilities as explanations for any new onset transaminase elevations, given that the patient had no evidence of liver disease at the onset of drug therapy [1,2,7]. These possibilities include (1) viral hepatitis: consider testing for hepatitis A, B, and C; (2) ethanol intake: the mean corpuscular volume and γ-glutamyl transpeptidase levels may support the role of ethanol in the process, when patient reliability is in question; (3) the presence of fatty liver changes in patients who are at least moderately obese (see below); and (4) an interaction with the specific dermatologic drug and a newly added drug from any prescriber source.

Management options for drug-induced hepatotoxicity

Overall, the key steps of management are to (1) stop the drug in question, (2) monitor appropriate LFTs closely, (3) seek appropriate consultations, and (4) provide supportive care. Fortunately, most patients who are diagnosed early on through systematic monitoring have completely reversible liver pathology. Given patient awareness of key symptoms to report and systematic monitoring of the liver by established standards of care for various drugs, irreversible end-stage liver disease caused by systemic drugs for dermatologic indications should be exceedingly rare.

For less severe complications, such as abnormal mild-moderate transaminase values in the one- to twofold elevation range, the clinician typically has the following *options* (can do several options simultaneously): (1) lower the drug dose, (2) stop the drug in question temporarily, (3) perform more frequent laboratory monitoring, and (4) seek consultation from a trustworthy consultant. When in doubt, lean toward the conservative side of the decision-making process until the severity of the liver abnormality is clarified.

Specific monitoring protocols

Drugs at least occasionally inducing hepatic toxicity

The drugs commonly used in dermatology that present a significant risk of hepatic toxicity include the following groups:

(1) hepatocellular toxicity (common causes): azathioprine, dapsone, methotrexate (occurs less commonly than steatosis → fibrosis), and acitretin
(2) hepatocellular toxicity (relatively *uncommon* causes): chlorambucil, cyclophosphamide, mycophenolate mofetil, cyclosporine, isotretinoin, hydroxychloroquine, chloroquine, itraconazole, and fluconazole

(3) drug hypersensitivity syndrome: dapsone, azathioprine, and minocycline
(4) steatosis → fibrosis: methotrexate (also acitretin very rarely; liver biopsies not required for acitretin therapy)

Hepatocellular toxicity monitoring

It is essential in the first 2 to 3 months of therapy to order hepatic transaminases (AST/SGOT and ALT/SGPT) at least monthly. For drugs such as azathioprine, dapsone, and methotrexate for which hematologic monitoring is likely to be ordered every 2 weeks initially, it is practical to order one or both transaminases every time a CBC is ordered. In contrast, monthly testing at the outset is appropriate for acitretin. After the initial 2 to 3 months of therapy, the transaminase values can be decreased to testing every 2 to 3 months, provided that the drug dose is stable and the test results are normal. It is important to order the transaminases 2 weeks after a dose increase in these relatively high-risk drugs. Furthermore, abnormal test results necessitate more frequent testing (1 to 2 weeks apart) until a clear trend of the test results is established.

For drugs that are relatively uncommon causes of hepatocellular toxicity (group 2 under "Drugs at least occasionally causing toxicity") the ALT/SGOT and ALT/SGPT can be ordered at baseline, 1 month, and 3 months, then perhaps at 3- to 6-month intervals subsequently. Specifics of each drug's monitoring guidelines can be found in a recent textbook [24]. Subtle variations in the generalizations discussed above can be found as individual drugs are discussed in this book.

Drug hypersensitivity syndrome monitoring

The monitoring for DHS is identical to hepatocellular toxicity monitoring with one exception. Concomitant CBC values are pivotal to the diagnosis of this subset of hepatic toxicity. It is common for the absolute eosinophil count to exceed 1000/mm^3 and will rarely reach levels higher than 10,000/mm^3 in the presence of fulminant DHS. It is important to note that a characteristic morbilliform or erythrodermic cutaneous eruption is present concomitantly with symptoms resembling infectious mononucleosis (fever, fatigue, pharyngitis, and adenopathy). Patients receiving dapsone, azathioprine, and minocycline should be encouraged to report the above signs and symptoms promptly. Some authors suggest that with minocycline therapy, no laboratory monitoring is required unless the mononucleosis-like signs and symptoms are present [25].

Steatosis → fibrosis monitoring

This relatively unique category of hepatic toxicity primarily relates to methotrexate therapy in dermatology. The most recent guidelines concerning this risk still suggest a liver biopsy (preferably ultrasound guided) be performed no later than after a 1.5-g cumulative dose of methotrexate therapy, and subsequently after every 1.5 g of methotrexate [13]. Albeit not officially stated in the most recent monitoring guidelines, a delayed-baseline liver biopsy after 6 to 12 months of therapy is very reasonable once it is established that methotrexate is (1) well tolerated, (2) efficacious, and (3) needed for long-term therapy. In multiple studies it has been demonstrated that the various LFTs are neither adequately sensitive nor specific to replace the liver biopsy in the diagnosis of methotrexate-induced fibrosis and cirrhosis in psoriatic patients. The major controversies and complexities of methotrexate hepatic monitoring, including possible noninvasive tests of liver integrity, have been recently reviewed by Callen and colleagues [26].

Overview of hematologic toxicity

Hematologic toxicities from drugs used in dermatology are infrequent, but potentially life-threatening, adverse reactions. Awareness of possible hematologic adverse effects and their most likely timing of occurrence can direct appropriate monitoring for these important toxicities.

General principles

Mechanisms of hematologic toxicity

Hematologic toxicities have several primary mechanisms, including both toxic and immunologic etiologies [27]. In general, toxic reactions are insidious in onset, developing over weeks to months, although some toxic hematologic reactions may be seen earlier (ie, in days to weeks). With rechallenge, there is a latent period before onset of symptoms. On the other hand, immunologic reactions appear relatively early in the course of therapy. These reactions take days to weeks to develop and, once established, often follow a more explosive course. Immunologic reactions recur promptly after reexposure to even small doses of the causative agent [27]. A more comprehensive discussion on specifics of these two broad categories can be found in a recent chapter [28].

Timing of hematologic toxicity

The cytotoxic drugs used in dermatology, especially the antimetabolites (methotrexate and azathioprine) and alkylating agents (cyclophosphamide and chlorambucil), have leukopenia as their most common hematologic effect. Dapsone and sulfonamides likewise have relatively frequent hematologic toxicities.

The half-life of white blood cells (WBCs) is only 6 to 8 hours, compared with half-lives of 5 to 7 days and 60 days for platelets and red blood cells (RBCs), respectively. A fall in the WBC count often begins 5 to 14 days after administration of a cytotoxic agent [27]. Recovery of blood counts usually starts 7 to 10 days after cessation of drug use.

For the above drugs, agranulocytosis, hemolytic anemia, and thrombocytopenia are acute reactions most commonly occurring in the first month of therapy. In many cases, dapsone agranulocytosis occurs in the second or third month of therapy as well.

Prediction of risk for hematologic toxicities

The incidence of idiosyncratic reactions, whether attributable to genetics or random events, can be estimated from population studies. There are several large population studies of drug-related hematologic toxicity, although these studies have significant limitations [29–36]. Details of these studies are discussed in the following section.

Major categories of drug-induced hematologic toxicity

Agranulocytosis—selected studies

Agranulocytosis is defined as a neutrophil count of less than 500/mm [37]. It is often accompanied by fever, pharyngitis, dysphagia, and oral ulcerations. Mortality rate is approximately 10% (0% to 12%) [29–31] and is often secondary to septicemia. The drugs highlighted in studies reviewed in the following paragraph are limited to systemic drugs used commonly by dermatologists. Details on other drugs can be found in the full reference citations and a recent chapter [28].

Van der Klauw and colleagues [30] reviewed 206 cases of drug-associated agranulocytosis reported over a 20-year period (1974 to 1994) in the Netherlands. Among the most commonly implicated drugs were sulfasalazine, certain antibiotics (including trimethoprim-sulfamethoxazole and the penicillins), and cimetidine. A case-cohort study of 75 patients admitted to Dutch hospitals between 1987 and 1990 for drug-induced

agranulocytosis documented that trimethoprim-sulfamethoxazole was among the most commonly implicated drugs [32]. From a study performed in Saskatchewan, trimethoprim-sulfamethoxazole and beta-lactam antibiotics were commonly associated with agranulocytosis [33]. A study in Spain demonstrated agranulocytosis attributable to sulfonamides, beta-lactam antibiotics, and erythromycin [31]. A Swedish study looked at drug-induced hematologic toxicity over a 10-year period (1985 to 1994), with dapsone among the most common culprits ($65/10^6$ patient-years) [34].

Aplastic anemia (pancytopenia)

Aplastic anemia is defined by the presence of pancytopenia (hemoglobin <10 g/dL, neutrophil count $<1500/mm^3$, and platelet count $<100,000/mm^3$) with a hypocellular marrow [37]. Alternatively, aplastic anemia is defined by a hypocellular marrow with at least two of the following: (1) white blood count 3.5×10^9/L or lower, (2) platelet count 50×10^9/L or lower, and (3) hemoglobin concentration 100 g/L or lower (≤ 10 g/dL) [35]. The mortality rate of aplastic anemia is 46% [35]. A French group noted that colchicine was among the drugs associated with high risk of aplasia [36]. The Swedish Blood Dyscrasia study also found that 25% of their cases of aplastic anemia were probably drug-associated [34]. In this study, trimethoprim-sulfamethoxazole had a reported risk for pancytopenia of 13 cases/10^6 patient-years.

Thrombocytopenia

Thrombocytopenia is defined as a platelet count less than $100,000/mm^3$ [37]. In the northeastern United States, trimethoprim-sulfamethoxazole was among the drugs with the highest risk, causing 38 cases/1 million users per week. In a review of published case reports of drug-induced thrombocytopenia, sulfonamides were the most commonly implicated drugs [38]. Because this was not a case-control study, no relative risk ratio could be estimated. In the Swedish registry study, trimethoprim-sulfamethoxazole had a risk of 96 cases of thrombocytopenia per 10^6 patient-years [34]. The authors cautioned that concomitant viral illness might have been a confounding factor in a number of cases.

Drugs prescribed by dermatologists—risk of hematologic toxicity

Methotrexate

The primary etiology of methotrexate hematologic toxicity is through the drug's inhibition of dihydrofolate reductase. It follows that prophylactic administration of folic acid 1 to 5 mg daily may lessen toxicity, especially nausea, with minimal interference with efficacy [39]. Alternatively, folinic acid (leucovorin) 2.5 to 5 mg orally 24 hours after methotrexate administration can be used [40]. Higher doses of folinic acid ("Leucovorin rescue") may be used if more severe hematologic toxicity (agranulocytosis or pancytopenia) occurs.

Risk of cytopenias from methotrexate is greatest in the elderly, those with renal insufficiency, patients with hypoalbuminemia, and those who develop macrocytosis [41]. Cytopenias may occur as a late complication, even in patients on a stable dosage, particularly as the result of drug interactions involving methotrexate. The most notable late-onset interaction occurs with concomitant trimethoprim-sulfamethoxazole and methotrexate, although prophylactic doses of trimethoprim-sulfamethoxazole may not cause this reaction [42]. Trimethoprim also binds to dihydrofolate reductase, causing increased blockade of this enzyme. Sulfonamides can displace methotrexate from albumin, increasing the free drug's bioavailability.

Azathioprine

Azathioprine is a purine analog that is quickly converted to 6-mercaptopurine (6-MP), then subsequently metabolized by xanthine oxidase, thiopurine S-methyltransferase (TPMT), and hypoxanthine guanine phosphoribosyl transferase (HGPRT). Between 2% and 17% of patients develop hematologic toxicity, especially neutropenia [43]. Severe myelosuppression may be seen in patients with homozygous TPMT deficiency, which is transmitted as an autosomal-recessive trait and is found in 0.3% of the population, when studied in a predominantly white population [43,44]. Approximately 11% of individuals are heterozygotes who show intermediate activity of the enzyme, and present with a moderate risk of myelosuppression.

Pretreatment assays for TPMT activity help predict which patients would develop severe cytopenias, who would develop cumulative toxicity, and which group might be resistant to drug effect, requiring higher drug doses because of rapid metabolism of azathioprine to inactive metabolites [43,44].

Drug interaction between allopurinol and azathioprine or 6-MP is of particular importance. Inhibition of xanthine oxidase by allopurinol greatly enhances the myelotoxicity of these two antimetabolites, so it is prudent to avoid allopurinol in combination with azathioprine or 6-MP. However, if these two drugs must be used together, the *dose* of the antimetabolite or of allopurinol should be *reduced* by 75% [45].

Dapsone

There are three main hematologic toxicities of dapsone: hemolysis, methemoglobinemia, and agranulocytosis. This discussion will focus just on hemolysis and agranulocytosis risk. Once ingested, the drug undergoes N-hydroxylation. The resultant hydroxylamines appear to be responsible for the hematologic toxicities [46].

Patients with glucose-6-phosphate dehydrogenase (G6PD) deficiency are unable to reduce $NADP^+$ to NADPH at a normal rate and, thus, sustain brisk hemolysis from dapsone. A milder, or A-type, of G6PD deficiency usually occurs in African Americans, whereas a more severe form is seen in those of Mediterranean heritage. The Mediterranean form is not self-limited so the dapsone must be stopped to curb the hemolysis [47]. It is important to note that virtually all patients (regardless of G6PD status) have at least some degree of hemolysis that may reduce their hemoglobin levels by 1 to 2 g/dL with commonly used dapsone doses.

Dapsone-induced agranulocytosis is a relatively rare phenomenon. Population studies show an incidence of 65 cases/10^6 patient-years [34]. Agranulocytosis is most commonly seen between weeks 3 and 12 of treatment. Patients should be warned to seek treatment immediately if they develop fever, chills, pharyngitis, dysphagia, or oral ulcerations.

Sulfonamides

Sulfonamides have been associated with a variety of hematologic toxicities, including neutropenia, agranulocytosis, thrombocytopenia, and aplastic anemia [30–36]. Sulfasalazine has the greatest risk profile, but trimethoprim-sulfamethoxazole (TMP-SMX) is also responsible for a number of toxicities. This discussion will focus on TMP-SMX alone.

The Swedish adverse drug reaction supporting system found the incidence of any hematologic toxicity from TMP-SMX to be 1 case per 18,000 prescriptions [48]. The average treatment time with TMP-SMX before the diagnosis of agranulocytosis is 13 days in this database.

The relative risk of aplastic anemia from sulfonamides is low [35,36,49,50]. For TMP-SMX, the incidence of pancytopenia/aplastic anemia was 0.7 cases per million daily patient doses [49,50]. Special notice should be taken of the adverse drug interaction between methotrexate and TMP-SMX, which may result in pancytopenia [42].

Overall, however, studies of short-term and long-term (3 months) use of TMP-SMX found that adverse hematologic effects were infrequent, except in those patients with probable folic acid deficiency or those receiving higher than the usual dosages [51].

Cyclophosphamide

Cyclophosphamide is a potent immunosuppressive alkylating agent. Neutropenia occurs in 15% of rheumatology patients treated with cyclophosphamide [52]; however, unlike the occasional permanent aplasia seen with some of the other alkylating agents, marrow suppression from cyclophosphamide is typically reversible. Although thrombocytopenia may occur, cyclophosphamide is generally a platelet-sparing agent. Mesna (either oral or intravenous forms) may serve to prevent urologic toxicity when very high doses of cyclophosphamide are used, although this preventive measure is uncommonly used in dermatology.

Chlorambucil

Chlorambucil is also an alkylating agent. Myelosuppression commonly occurs with this drug as used in all of medicine, and occasionally may be profound or prolonged. Traditional dermatologic doses of 2 to 4 mg daily at the initiation of therapy typically produce relatively mild hematologic risk.

Antimalarials

Patients with G6PD deficiency have brisk hemolysis with primaquine, but are not at additional risk of hemolysis with the other more commonly used antimalarial agents (hydroxychloroquine, chloroquine, and quinacrine) when given at standard doses [53]. Leukopenia has been seen with each of the antimalarials, occurring in 4.8% of patients on chloroquine, but less frequently in those on hydroxychloroquine. Isolated cases of agranulocytosis have been noted with all the antimalarial agents, including a patient on hydroxychloroquine who received an extremely high dose.

Colchicine

Hematologic toxicity is generally associated with acute drug overdose [54], but has been described with therapeutic doses during acute or chronic therapy [55,56]. The risk is higher for patients with renal or hepatic insufficiency [56] and in those patients receiving intravenous colchicine [57].

Mycophenolate mofetil

Mycophenolate mofetil is a relatively new immunosuppressive drug that inhibits de novo purine synthesis in stimulated T cells and B cells by blocking the enzyme type II inosine monophosphate dehydrogenase [58,59]. Occasional hematologic toxicities occur, including relatively infrequent leukopenia, anemia, and thrombocytopenia [40,58,59].

Efalizumab and infliximab

In the initial studies of efalizumab, thrombocytopenia occurred in 0.3% of treated patients, usually appearing at 2 to 6 months [60]. Platelet counts recovered in seven of eight patients; the eighth patient was lost to follow up. Agranulocytosis attributable to infliximab is very uncommon [61].

Systemic retinoids

Mild neutropenia may occur relatively often with the oral retinoids isotretinoin and acitretin, but agranulocytosis is exceedingly rare [62].

Terbinafine

Terbinafine has been associated with agranulocytosis in at least four patients [63–65]. The agranulocytosis occurred after 4 to 6 weeks of therapy. The estimated incidence is 1 in 400,000 patients [64].

Treatment of hematologic toxicities

Guidelines for drug cessation and rechallenge

Reductions of drug dose should be considered for a new neutropenia of 1500 to 2000/mm^3 or leukopenia of 3000 to 3500/mm^3 (Table 3). Cessation of the drug in question should be considered for a new neutropenia of less than 1500/mm^3, or for thrombocytopenia of less than 100,000/mm^3. A suspect drug should definitely be stopped when the neutrophil count falls below 1000/mm^3 or the platelet count below 50,000/mm^3 [27].

Management of agranulocytosis

Fever in a patient with an absolute neutrophil count of less than 500/mm^3 is a medical emergency and should be immediately treated in a hospital setting with broad-spectrum antibiotic coverage pending results of cultures. Recombinant human granulocyte colony–stimulating factors, including pegfilgrastim, have been used to

Table 3
General guidelines for drug discontinuation for cytopenias (cell count per μL)

Cellular subset	Reduce drug dose (at a minimum)	Strongly consider discontinuing drug	Definitely stop the drug in question
White blood cells	3000–3500	2500–3000	<2500
Granulocytes	1500–2000	1000–1500	<1000
Platelets	100,000–150,000	50,000–100,000	<50,000

These are rough guidelines; each clinical scenario should be handled individually. Of particular importance is the rate of change and the timing of the change.

Data from Hande KR. Principles and pharmacology of chemotherapy. In: Lee RG, Foerster J, Lukens JN, et al, editors. Wintrobe's clinical hematology. Vol. 2. 10th edition. Baltimore (MD): Lippincott Williams & Wilkins; 1999. p. 2085.

help reverse drug-induced neutropenia. Other agents, such as intravenous immune globulin (0.4 mg/kg daily × 5 days), also have been used to treat drug-induced immune thrombocytopenia and agranulocytosis [66].

Specific approaches to hematologic toxicity monitoring

Some background issues

The drugs discussed in this section on hematologic toxicity can be divided into several major categories. These categories include drugs presenting the risk of agranulocytosis, pancytopenia, or both:

(1) Relatively high-risk drugs: methotrexate, azathioprine, dapsone, cyclophosphamide, and chlorambucil
(2) Relatively low-risk drugs: sulfonamides, antimalarials, colchicine, mycophenolate mofetil, infliximab, retinoids, and terbinafine

In addition several subcategories can be derived from the concepts discussed in this chapter. These subcategories include the following:

(1) Drugs with unique risk of hemolysis: dapsone
(2) Drugs with unique risk of thrombocytopenia: sulfonamides and efalizumab

Specific monitoring protocols

Relatively high-risk drugs for hematologic toxicity: agranulocytosis and pancytopenia

Detailed specific monitoring guidelines for the great majority of the above drugs can be found in a recent textbook [24]. In this article, we will attempt to provide the key concepts behind the specific guidelines.

In general, when administering relatively high-risk drugs, one should order a CBC with differential and platelets at least every 2 weeks during the time of greatest likelihood for hematologic toxicities, that is, the first 2 to 3 months. Weekly monitoring of the CBC is often suggested during the first month of therapy with some drugs, such as cyclophosphamide or chlorambucil. These protocols would be appropriate as long as the total WBC is at least 3500 to 4000/mm³ and neutrophil count is at least 2000/mm³. More frequent monitoring and drug dosage reduction are generally necessary for a total WBC of 3000 to 3500/mm³ and/or neutrophil count of 1500 to 2000/mm³. Most would suggest following the CBC at least weekly with WBC and/or neutrophil counts in this latter range. It is important to factor in the rate of decline as well. Even when the WBC/neutrophil counts reside in the normal range, if the fall in values was rapid or steep, it is advisable to check a CBC within a week to further establish the trend of the decline. Furthermore, with rapidly decreasing "counts," stopping the drug in question until the trend of the lab values is clarified is appropriate.

After 2 to 3 months of therapy and with stable drug dosages, these relatively high-risk drugs may be monitored much less frequently. Clinicians may gradually increase the time between laboratory tests from 2-week intervals to 6- to 8-week intervals over the subsequent 3 months. However, if the drug dose is raised beyond that used in the initial 3 months of therapy, it is suggested the clinician order a CBC to be drawn within 2 weeks following the dose increase.

Two specific points need to be made concerning methotrexate hematologic monitoring. First, the lab testing should always be done 5 to 6 days after the weekly methotrexate dose to avoid overconcern regarding the expected decrease in

WBC/neutrophils in the days immediately following methotrexate intake. Second, a so-called "test dose" for methotrexate is used primarily to uncover any rapid, unexpected hematologic toxicity with the first dose of the drug. In this case, it is appropriate to order a CBC a week after the first dose, then to decrease testing to 2-week intervals.

Relatively low-risk drugs for hematologic toxicity: agranulocytosis and pancytopenia

With prolonged use of drugs in this group, patients should have a baseline CBC followed by retesting 4 to 6 weeks after initiation of therapy. Long-term therapy should be monitored quarterly for the first 6 to 12 months, then perhaps semiannually. However, if there are no hematologic toxicities uncovered in the first 2 to 3 months, it is very uncommon to see test result changes subsequently.

For colchicine therapy, retesting a CBC monthly for the first 3 months is appropriate, whereas for the other drugs in this relatively low-risk drug category the above protocol is sufficient. Many clinicians do not routinely do hematologic testing for sulfonamides (specifically TMP-SMX) when prescribed long term for severe acne or hidradenitis. Given the relatively frequent presence of this drug family in the list of medications commonly inducing either agranulocytosis or pancytopenia in multiple studies cited earlier, it is wise to order a baseline CBC with follow-up testing 1 to 2 times in the first several months of therapy, then at least yearly.

Drugs with a unique risk of hemolysis

This category primarily includes dapsone. The unique test to add to the laboratory monitoring armamentarium is the reticulocyte count. Following the reticulocyte count with each CBC provides a barometer of sorts for the degree of hemolysis. Reticulocyte counts in the range of 4% to 8% suggests a substantial degree of hemolysis is occurring and that dapsone dose increases from this point forward should be done very cautiously. A falling reticulocyte count (when previously in this range) strongly suggests that the body is becoming deficient of nutrients (iron, B_{12}, and folate) important to RBC production. This is particularly true if the hemoglobin level is falling simultaneously.

There have been four reports of hemolytic anemia during therapy with efalizumab, generally occurring around 4 to 6 months. No specific monitoring for this complication is indicated beyond the CBC obtained to monitor platelet levels.

Drugs with a unique risk of thrombocytopenia

Based on the epidemiologic studies cited earlier, this category includes primarily efalizumab and the sulfonamides. Rarely, patients receiving methotrexate have an isolated decrease in the platelet count. Overall, the risk of clinically important thrombocytopenia ($<50,000$ platelets/mm^3) is very uncommon with any of these drugs. Routinely requesting that the platelet count be ordered with the CBC suffices in the surveillance for isolated thrombocytopenia for the drugs discussed in this chapter.

References

[1] Zimmerman HJ, Ishak KG. General aspects of drug-induced liver disease. Gastroenterol Clin North Am 1995;24:739–57.

[2] Lee WM. Medical progress: drug-induced hepatotoxicity. N Engl J Med 2003;349:474–85.

[3] O'Grady JG, Alexander GJ, Hayllar KM, et al. Early indicators of prognosis in fulminant hepatic failure. Gastroenterology 1989;97:439–45.

[4] Walgren JL, Mitchell MD, Thompson DC. Role of metabolism in drug-induced idiosyncratic hepatotoxicity. Crit Rev Toxicol 2005;35:325–61.

[5] Fontana RJ, Watkins PB. Genetic predisposition to drug-induced liver disease. Gastroenterol Clin North Am 1995;24:811–37.

[6] Pessayre D. Role of reactive metabolites in drug-induced hepatitis. J Hepatol 1995;23(Suppl 1):16–24.

[7] Van Pelt FN, Straub P, Manns MP. Molecular basis of drug-induced immunological liver injury. Semin Liver Dis 1995;15:283–300.

[8] Robin MA, LeRoy M, Descatoire V, et al. Plasma membrane cytochromes P450 as neoantigens and autoimmune targets in drug-induced hepatitis. J Hepatol 1997;26(Suppl 1):23–30.

[9] Beaune PH, Bourdi M. Autoantibodies against cytochromes P-450 in drug-induced autoimmune hepatitis. Ann N Y Acad Sci 1993;685:641–5.

[10] Seeff LB, Cuccherini BA, Zimmerman HJ, et al. Acetaminophen hepatotoxicity in alcoholics: a therapeutic misadventure. Ann Intern Med 1986; 104:399–404.

[11] Lee WM. Medical progress: drug-induced hepatotoxicity. N Engl J Med 1995;333:1118–27.

[12] Garibaldi RA, Drusin RE, Ferebee SH, et al. Isoniazid-associated hepatitis: report of an outbreak. Am Rev Respir Dis 1972;106:357–65.

[13] Roenigk HH Jr, Auerbach R, Maibach HI, et al. Methotrexate in psoriasis: consensus conference. J Am Acad Dermatol 1998;38:478–85.

[14] Wolverton SE. Major adverse effects from systemic drugs: defining the risks. Curr Probl Dermatol 1995;7:1–40.

[15] Vahlquist A. Long-term safety of retinoid therapy. J Am Acad Dermatol 1992;27:S29–33.

[16] Knowles SR, Gupta AK, Shear NH, et al. Azathioprine hypersensitivity-like reactions—a case report and a review of the literature. Clin Exp Dermatol 1995;20:353–6.

[17] Prussick R, Shear NH. Dapsone hypersensitivity syndrome. J Am Acad Dermatol 1996;35:346–9.

[18] Lawrence WA, Olsen HW, Nickles DJ. Dapsone hepatitis. Arch Intern Med 1987;147:175.

[19] Elkayam O, Yaron M, Caspi D. Minocycline-induced autoimmune syndromes: an overview. Semin Arthritis Rheum 1999;28:392–7.

[20] Knowles S, Shapiro L, Shear N. Serious adverse reactions induced by minocycline: a report of 13 patients and review of the literature. Arch Dermatol 1996;132:934–9.

[21] Tygstrup N. Assessment of liver function: principles and practice. J Gastroenterol Hepatol 1990;5:468–82.

[22] Sallie R, Tredger JM, Williams R. Drugs and the liver. Part 1: testing liver function. Biopharm Drug Dispos 1991;12:251–9.

[23] Giannini EG, Testa R, Savarino V. Liver enzyme alteration: a guide for clinicians. CMAJ 2005;172:367–79.

[24] Wolverton SE, editor. Comprehensive dermatologic drug therapy. 2nd edition. London: Elsevier; 2007.

[25] Knowles SR, Shear NH. Cutaneous drug reactions with systemic features. In: Wolverton SE, editor. Comprehensive dermatologic drug therapy. 2nd edition. London: Elsevier; 2007. p. 977–88.

[26] Callen JP, Kulp-Shorten CL, Wolverton SE. Methotrexate. In: Wolverton SE, editor. Comprehensive dermatologic drug therapy. 2nd edition. London: Elsevier; 2007. p. 163–81.

[27] Verweij J, Sparreboom A, Nooter K. Antitumor antibiotics. In: Chabner BA, Longo DL, editors. Cancer chemotherapy and biotherapy. 3rd edition. Philadelphia: Lippincott Williams & Wilkins; 2001. p. 490.

[28] Remlinger KA. Hematologic toxicity of drug therapy. In: Wolverton SE, editor. Comprehensive dermatologic drug therapy. 2nd edition. London: Elsevier; 2007. p. 893–909.

[29] van Staa TP, Boulton F, Cooper C, et al. Neutropenia and agranulocytosis in England and Wales: incidence and risk factors. Am J Hematol 2003;72:248–54.

[30] van der Klauw MM, Wilson JHP, Stricker BHC. Drug-associated agranulocytosis: 20 years of reporting in the Netherlands (1974–1994). Am J Hematol 1998;57:206–11.

[31] Ibanez L, Vidal X, Ballarin E, et al. Population-based drug-induced agranulocytosis. Arch Intern Med 2005;165:869–74.

[32] van der Klauw MM, Goudsmit R, Halie R, et al. A population-based case-cohort study of drug-associated agranulocytosis. Arch Intern Med 1999;159:369–74.

[33] Rawson NB, Harding SR, Malcolm E, et al. Hospitalizations for aplastic anemia and agranulocytosis in Saskatchewan: incidence and associations with antecedent prescription drug use. J Clin Epidemiol 1998;12:1345–55.

[34] Wiholm B-E, Emanuelsson S. Drug-related blood dyscrasias in a Swedish reporting system, 1985–1994. Eur J Haematol 1996;57(Suppl):42–6.

[35] Kaufman DW, Kelly JP, Jurgelon JM, et al. Drugs in the aetiology of agranulocytosis and aplastic anaemia. Eur J Haematol 1996;57(Suppl):23–30.

[36] Baumelou E, Guiguet M, Mary JY, et al. Epidemiology of aplastic anemia in France: a case control study. I. Medical history and medication use. Blood 1993;81:1471–8.

[37] Standardization of definitions and criteria of causality assessment of adverse drug reactions. Drug-induced cytopenia. Int J Clin Pharmacol Ther Toxicol 1991;29:75–81.

[38] George JN, Raskob GE, Shah SR, et al. Drug-induced thrombocytopenia: a systematic review of published case reports. Ann Intern Med 1998;129:886–90.

[39] Duhra P. Treatment of gastrointestinal symptoms associated with methotrexate therapy for psoriasis. J Am Acad Dermatol 1993;28:466–9.

[40] Silvis NG. Antimetabolites and cytotoxic drugs. Dermatol Clin 2001;19:105–18.

[41] Weinblatt ME, Fraser P. Elevated mean corpuscular volume as a predictor of hematologic toxicity due to methotrexate therapy. Arthritis Rheum 1989;32:1592–6.

[42] Andersen WK, Feingold DS. Adverse drug interactions clinically important for the dermatologist. Arch Dermatol 1995;131:468–73.

[43] Anstey A. Azathioprine in dermatology: a review in light of advances in understanding methylation pharmacogenetics. J R Soc Med 1995;88(Suppl):155P–60P.

[44] Anstey AV, Wakelin S, Reynolds NJ. Guidelines for prescribing azathioprine in dermatology. Br J Dermatol 2004;151:1123–32.

[45] Hande KR. Purine antimetabolites. In: Chabner BA, Longo DL, editors. Cancer chemotherapy and biotherapy. 3rd edition. Philadelphia: Lippincott Williams & Wilkins; 2001. p. 295–308.

[46] Coleman MD. Dapsone-mediated agranulocytosis: risks, possible mechanisms and prevention. Toxicology 2001;162:53–60.

[47] Gregg XT, Prchal JT, et al. Red blood cells: enzymopathies of glutathione metabolism. In: Hoffman R, Benz EJ, Shattil SJ, editors. Hematology: basic principles and practice. 4th edition. Philadelphia: Elsevier; 2004. p. 657–60.

[48] Keisu M, Wiholm B-E, Palmblad J. Trimethoprim-sulphamethoxazole-associated blood dyscrasias. Ten years' experience of the Swedish spontaneous reporting system. J Intern Med 1990;228:353–60.

[49] Mary JY, Guiget M, Baumelou E, et al. Drug use and aplastic anaemia: the French experience. Eur J Haematol 1996;57(Suppl):35–41.

[50] Anttila PM, Valimaki M, Pentikainen PJ. Pure-red-cell aplasia associated with sulphasalazine but not 5-aminosalicylic acid [letter]. Lancet 1985;2:1006.

[51] Herbert V. Metabolism of folic acid in man. J Infect Dis 1973;128(Suppl):S601–6.

[52] Grove ML, Hassell AB, Hay EM, et al. Adverse reactions to disease-modifying anti-rheumatic drugs in clinical practice. QJM 2001;94:309–19.

[53] Beutler E. The hemolytic effect of primaquine and related compounds: a review. Blood 1959;14:103–39.

[54] Ben-Chetrit E, Levy M. Colchicine: 1998 update. Semin Arthritis Rheum 1998;28:48–59.

[55] Dixon AJ, Wall GC. Probable colchicine-induced neutropenia not related to intentional overdose. Ann Pharmacother 2001;35:192–5.

[56] Ferrannini E, Pentimone F. Marrow aplasia following colchicine treatment for gouty arthritis. Clin Exp Rheumatol 1984;2:173–5.

[57] Ducloux D, Schuller V, Chalopin J-M. Colchicine agranulocytosis [letter]. Nephrol Dial Transplant 1997;12:1541–2.

[58] Grundmann-Kollmann M, Korting HC, Behrens S, et al. Mycophenolate mofetil: a new therapeutic option in the treatment of blistering autoimmune diseases. J Am Acad Dermatol 1999;40:957–60.

[59] Enk AH, Knop J. Mycophenolate is effective in the treatment of pemphigus vulgaris. Arch Dermatol 1999;135:54–6.

[60] Raptiva® (efalizumab) [package insert]. South San Francisco (CA): Genentech; 2003.

[61] Favalli EG, Varenna M, Sinigaglia L. Drug-induced agranulocytosis during treatment with infliximab in enteropathic spondyloarthropathy. Clin Exp Rheumatol 2005;23:247–50.

[62] Windhorst DB, Nigra T. General clinical toxicology of oral retinoids. J Am Acad Dermatol 1982;6:675–82.

[63] Kovacs MJ, Alshammari S, Guenther L, et al. Neutropenia and pancytopenia associated with oral terbinafine [letter]. J Am Acad Dermatol 1994;31:806.

[64] Gupta AK, Soori GS, Del Rosso JQ, et al. Severe neutropenia associated with oral terbinafine therapy. J Am Acad Dermatol 1998;38:765–7.

[65] Ornstein DL, Ely P. Reversible agranulocytosis associated with oral terbinafine for onychomycosis. J Am Acad Dermatol 1998;39:1023–4.

[66] Salama A, Mueller-Eckhardt C. Immune-mediated blood cell dyscrasias related to drugs. Semin Hematol 1992;29:54–63.

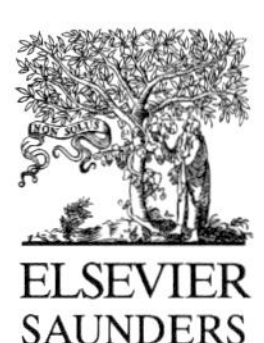

ELSEVIER
SAUNDERS

Dermatol Clin 25 (2007) 207–213

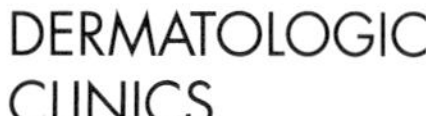

DERMATOLOGIC
CLINICS

Potential Complications Associated with the Use of Biologic Agents for Psoriasis

Joshua A. Zeichner, MD, Mark Lebwohl, MD*

Department of Dermatology, Mount Sinai Medical Center, 5 East 98th Street, Box 1048,
New York, NY 10029, USA

Psoriasis is a chronic, remitting, and relapsing inflammatory disease affecting the skin. The joints may also be involved in the form of psoriatic arthritis. Disease manifestations vary in severity, and severe forms may significantly impair patients' quality of life. The goal of psoriasis treatment is to gain rapid control of the disease process and to maintain long-term remissions. Mild cases may be treated with topical preparations, such as corticosteroids, vitamin D analogs, and retinoids. Moderate and severe psoriasis often requires phototherapy or systemic therapies, including methotrexate, acitretin, cyclosporine, or biologic agents. Treatment regimens may be tailored to meet the specific needs and preferences of each patient.

There is no cure for psoriasis, and patients often require some form of therapy to sustain remission. The side-effect profiles of particular medicines may limit the long-term use, however. Traditional systemic therapies, such as methotrexate, cyclosporine, and acitretin, are effective but may not be tolerated by all patients. Liver toxicity is a serious risk that increases with the total cumulative dose of methotrexate. Therefore, it is recommended that patients on long-term methotrexate therapy undergo periodic liver biopsies for monitoring [1]. Additionally, nausea, upset stomach, lethargy, and bone marrow toxicity are associated with methotrexate [2]. Cyclosporine is nephrotoxic and may lead to hypertension [3,4]. Patients on acitretin commonly experience dose-dependent xerosis and cheilitis and are often maintained on long-term, low-dose therapy (≤ 25 mg daily), as high doses are more likely to cause side effects and elevations in serum lipids [5]. Acitretin is teratogenic, so it should be avoided in women of childbearing potential [6].

The biologic agents have added greatly to the armamentarium of psoriasis medications. The drugs in this class have each been engineered to target a specific step in the inflammatory cascade that leads to psoriasis. These medications may be subcategorized as either inhibitors of T-cell activity or as cytokine antagonists [7,8]. The cytokine antagonists include the tumor necrosis factor alpha (TNF-α) inhibitors etanercept, infliximab, and adalimumab. T-cell blocking agents include efalizumab and alefacept. While these new medications are generally safe and effective, both physicians and patients must understand the potential risks and side effects associated with each of them.

Tumor necrosis factor alpha antagonists

TNF-α is a pro-inflammatory cytokine produced by T-cell lymphocytes, macrophages, and keratinocytes, and has been found at high levels in psoriatic skin [9]. It stimulates the production of other cytokines, including interleukin-1 (IL-1), IL-6, and IL-8; up-regulates the transcription factor nuclear factor kappa beta; and promotes keratinocyte proliferation. All of these signals may lead to pathologic inflammation in several organs, such as skin and joints. Through TNF-α neutralization, antagonist medications disrupt the inflammatory cascade central to the pathophysiology of psoriasis and psoriatic arthritis [9,10].

Etanercept

Etanercept is a soluble fusion protein composed of the p75 subunit of the TNF-α receptor

---

* Corresponding author.

E-mail address: lebwohl@aol.com (M. Lebwohl).

and the Fc portion of human IgGl [11,12]. The drug is a dimer and has a greater affinity for TNF-α than the body's naturally occurring monomeric receptors [11,13]. Etanercept competitively binds TNF-α and prevents binding to endogenous receptors, thereby inhibiting the ensuing inflammatory cascade associated with the pathogenesis of psoriasis [13]. Etanercept is approved by the U.S. Food and Drug Administration to treat rheumatoid arthritis, juvenile rheumatoid arthritis, ankylosing spondilitis, psoriatic arthritis, and psoriasis. Administration is through weekly or biweekly subcutaneous injections.

Injection site reactions are the most commonly reported adverse events associated with etanercept. During clinical trials, approximately 14% of psoriasis patients developed erythema, pruritus, pain, or swelling at sites of injection [14]. These were generally mild to moderate and occurred within the first few months of therapy. Injection site reactions tended to become less frequent after using the drug for several months, and this complication generally did not lead to discontinuation of the drug [15].

As with all immunosuppressive medications, etanercept carries the risk of infection. Infections were common in clinical trials for both rheumatoid arthritis and psoriasis, but rates were similar in patients on etanercept and on placebo. Upper respiratory tract infections were the most frequent type of infection, occurring in 20% of rheumatoid arthritis patients and 12% of psoriasis patients. Serious infections were uncommon, and many of the patients who developed serious infections had underlying predisposing medical conditions [14]. Rare infections, including *Histoplasma capsulatum* and *Listeria monocytogenes* [16–18], have been reported in the literature. These infections have occurred more often in patients on anti-TNF antibodies than in those treated with such fusion protein receptor drugs as etanercept. Regardless, in the event of a serious infection, the drug should be withheld.

Physicians prescribing anti-TNF drugs must consider the risk for development of active tuberculosis through either reactivation of latent disease or a new infection. TNF-α plays a key role in granuloma formation through macrophage activation [19–21]. This helps to explain the high percentage of extrapulmonary or disseminated cases of tuberculosis occurring in patients on anti-TNF therapy. In the case of infliximab, up to 65% of reported cases of tuberculosis are extrapulmonary, compared with 15% to 25% in the

general population [22]. In etanercept-treated patients, there has been no significant increase in the risk of reactivation of tuberculosis [8,14]. Tuberculin skin testing before initiation of therapy is prudent, and results should be evaluated in the context of the patient's personal history, according to the Centers for Disease Control and Prevention guidelines [23]. The medical evaluation of all patients with a positive tuberculin skin test should include a chest radiograph. Currently, there are no recommendations for tuberculosis prophylaxis in the package inserts for the biologic agents. However, the Centers for Disease Control and Prevention's preferred therapy for tuberculosis prophylaxis is isoniazid 5 mg/kg (maximum of 300 mg) daily for 9 months. Patients should also receive supplemental vitamin B6 [23–25].

It is unclear whether TNF-α inhibition increases the risk of lymphoma [26]. At baseline, patients with autoimmune diseases like psoriasis are more likely to develop lymphoproliferative diseases than the general population [27,28]. Additionally, chronic inflammation and previous immunosuppressive medications are independent risk factors [26]. In clinical trials, the overall risk of malignancy was not increased by etanercept in rheumatoid arthritis patients [29]. However, cases of lymphomas have been reported in patients on etanercept, and some of these resolved after discontinuation of the drug [30].

Both peripheral and central demyelinating disorders, including multiple sclerosis, have been reported to develop in patients taking TNF-α antagonists [14,29,31–33]. These medications should be avoided in the setting of a personal or family history of demyelinating conditions. There are reports of patients with new-onset neurologic symptoms that improved after the biologic agent was stopped [33]. Onset of new neurological symptoms in a patient on TNF-α inhibitors that suggest the development of a demyelinating disorder should be promptly evaluated and the drug should be withheld.

The issue of prescribing etanercept and other TNF-α blockers in patients with congestive heart failure (CHF) is controversial. Two large studies evaluating the use of etanercept in New York Heart Association congestive heart failure (classes II–IV) were terminated early due to lack of efficacy [34]. These were the Randomized Etanercept North American Strategy to Study Antagonism of Cytokines trial, also known as the Renaissance trial, and the Research into Etanercept: Cytokine Antagonism in Ventricular

Dysfunction trial, also known as the Recover trial. Additionally, the Randomized Etanercept Worldwide Evaluation, the so-called "Renewal" evaluation of the Renaissance and Recover trials, showed no benefit on mortality or CHF morbidity [35]. However, there is some evidence that TNF-α blockade is of benefit to the failing heart. A 2004 report showed that the incidence of CHF in rheumatoid arthritis patients on anti-TNF medications (either infliximab or etanercept) was significantly lower than in those not on these medicines (3.1% compared with 3.8%) [36]. Moreover, another study demonstrated a dose-dependent improvement in both left ventricular function and structure in CHF patients on etanercept [37]. At present, until more data is accumulated, etanercept and the other TNF-α inhibitors should be prescribed with caution to patients with a preexisting diagnosis or risk factors for development of CHF.

Infliximab

Infliximab is a monoclonal antibody that competitively binds both soluble and membrane-bound forms of TNF-α. The drug is chimeric, comprised of a human IgG1 constant region and murine variable regions specific for TNF-α [38]. Infliximab is indicated for the treatment of psoriatic arthritis, Crohn's disease, ankylosing spondylitis, and rheumatoid arthritis, and is administered as an intravenous infusion.

The most common adverse events from infliximab are infusion-related reactions, defined as events occurring during or immediately following the intravenous infusion. Reactions include urticaria, fever, blood pressure fluctuation, and, uncommonly, anaphylaxis. Twenty percent of patients in clinical trials developed an infusion reaction, versus 10% of patients receiving placebo [38]. Patients are commonly premedicated with an antihistamine and an antipyretic before administration and should be frequently monitored during the infusion.

As an immunosuppressive agent, infection is a major concern in patients on infliximab, as it is for the other TNF-α inhibitors. Rheumatoid arthritis patients on anti-TNF antibodies including infliximab and adalimumab have been shown to be at an increased risk to develop an infection [39]. Patients with chronic or recurring infections should be prescribed the drug cautiously, and it should be discontinued in the event of a serious infection [40]. Thirty-six percent of infliximab

patients developed infections in clinical trials, compared with 25% in the placebo arm [38]. Reactivation of latent tuberculosis and the potential to develop new infection is a concern in patients on infliximab, more so than with etanercept [38,41]. Prior to starting infliximab therapy, all patients must be properly evaluated with a tuberculin skin test and a chest radiograph, if indicated. A latent infection must be treated prophylactically [25].

Other potential side effects of infliximab are similar to those of etanercept. Demyelinating diseases may be unmasked or exacerbated [29,33], so the medication should not be prescribed to patients with a history of central or peripheral demyelinating disorders. Also, CHF has not been shown to improve in patients on TNF-α blockers [42]. Finally, a recent study has demonstrated a dose-dependent risk of developing a malignancy in rheumatoid arthritis patients on anti-TNF antibody medication. Included in the report were blood cell, skin, and solid organ tumors [39]. However, in the case of lymphomas, a causal relationship has not been established with infliximab [30].

Several rare but potentially serious conditions are associated with infliximab. Patients have been reported to develop liver toxicity, manifesting as hepatitis, acute liver failure, jaundice, or cholestasis. In most of these cases, patients were also exposed to a hepatotoxic drug, so the association is unclear. Regardless, any patients developing a significant elevation of their liver enzymes or clinical signs of hepatotoxicity, such as jaundice, should be evaluated and infliximab therapy should be discontinued [38]. Additionally, hematologic abnormalities may be associated with infliximab. Leukopenia, neutropenia, thrombocytopenia, and pancytopenia have been reported and should be considered in patients developing pallor, easy bruising, bleeding, or fever.

Adalimumab

Adalimumab is a humanized, monoclonal antibody targeting TNF-α. Administered as a biweekly subcutaneous injection, the drug is approved for the treatment of rheumatoid and psoriatic arthritis. Adalimumab is the newest of the drugs in its class, and available safety data are limited. As a general rule, practitioners should take the same precautions with this drug as they do with etanercept and infliximab.

Common side effects include injection site reactions in up to 20% of patients [43]. As with the other anti-TNF antibody, infliximab, a dose-dependent increase in malignancy risk has been observed when adalimumab is used in rheumatoid arthritis patients [39]. While an increased infection risk has been reported in one recent meta-analysis [39], in the 24-week long Safety Trial of Adalimumab in Rheumatoid Arthritis study, known as the Star study, adalimumab used in conjunction with standard rheumatoid arthritis medications did not result in a predisposition for infection [44]. Finally, the same caution for developing lymphoproliferative disorders, demyelinating diseases, and heart failure must be taken before adalimumab administration [30].

Anti–T-cell agents

Psoriasis is an immune-mediated disease characterized by overactive T lymphocytes. Abnormal cytokine production leads to a complex inflammatory cascade that drives T-cell activation and migration. Psoriatic plaques are characterized by keratinocyte hyperproliferation and an abundance of both CD4+ and CD8+ T cells [45]. Many psoriasis medications therefore target T cells and inhibit their activity. Drugs in this category include cyclosporine and the biologic agents, efalizumab and alefacept.

Efalizumab

Efalizumab is a humanized, monoclonal antibody that targets the T-cell surface protein lymphocyte function associated antigen-1 (LFA-1). Specifically, efalizumab binds CDlla, the α-subunit of LFA-1 [46]. The drug blocks the interaction between LFA-1 and intracellular adhesion molecule-1 on endothelial surfaces. Efalizumab thereby inhibits the pathologic activation and migration of T cells to the skin [47,48]. Administered as a subcutaneous injection, the medication is approved for moderate to severe psoriasis.

The first dose of efalizumab is commonly accompanied by adverse reactions, which include headaches, nausea, chills, and fevers. This has been reported in 29% of patients and may be observed during the first few days of treatment [49]. The reactions typically disappear by the third dose, and premedication with acetaminophen may be useful. Additionally, clinical trial data show 29% of patients develop nonspecific infections, which is not statistically higher than that of the placebo group, in which 26% developed nonspecific infections [50]. Efalizumab treatment should be discontinued in the case of a serious infection.

Rare instances of psoriasis exacerbation have been reported in patients on efalizumab. Though uncommon, worsening of the disease during treatment may be severe, and psoriasis can convert from a plaque to a pustular type. Both new-onset and deterioration of preexisting arthritis has also been observed in efalizumab-treated patients in clinical trials, though infrequently [49].

Hematologic abnormalities, including anemia and thrombocytopenia, have been observed in patients on efalizumab. Thrombocytopenia has been reported in 0.3% of patients on the drug in clinical trials. As a result, periodic platelet counts are required of patients throughout their treatment [49].

Efalizumab treatment must not be abruptly terminated, as there is an association with rebound psoriasis after rapid discontinuation of the drug. Disease rebound, defined as either 25% Psoriasis Assessment and Severity Index (PASI) score worsening from pretreatment baseline or as a change in psoriasis form, may occur in up to 13.4% of patients who end treatment abruptly [49]. A rebound may require hospitalization for treatment and may manifest as pustular, guttate, or erythrodermic psoriasis [51]. To transition a patient off efalizumab safely, physicians should overlap another agent with efalizumab for several weeks before discontinuing the drug. In doing so, the risk for a flare may be avoided.

Patients on efalizumab have not been found to be at an increased risk to develop a malignancy. However, because efalizumab is an immunomodulator, caution should be taken in combining it with other immunosuppressive medications [49].

Alefacept

Alefacept is an LFA-3–IgG1 fusion protein that targets the CD2 protein on the surface of T lymphocytes. Alefacept blocks binding of endogenous LFA-3 and the resulting T-cell activation and proliferation [48,52]. The drug also induces apoptosis of T cells with high levels of CD2 through aggregation with FcγRIII IgG receptors on natural killer cells and macrophages [53,54]. Alefacept therefore decreases the number of circulating CD45RO+ T lymphocytes, which are key players in the pathophysiology of psoriasis [53,55]. Alefacept was the first biologic agent approved for psoriasis and is administered as a weekly intramuscular injection.

As with the other injected biologic agents, injection site reactions are common. Sixteen percent of patients in clinical trials reported pain and inflammation after injection. These reactions were generally mild and did not result in discontinuation from the study [56,57]. Other reported side effects include pharyngitis, dizziness, cough, nausea, pruritus, muscle aches, and chills. Only chills occurred at a higher rate in the alefacept-treated patients (6%) compared with the placebo (1%) [56].

Lymphopenia is common in patients on alefacept, and is potentially dangerous if levels fall too low. Before initiation of treatment, patients must have baseline blood counts taken. Their CD4+ levels should be normal at baseline and frequently monitored while on alefacept [56]. The drug should be discontinued if CD4+ T-cell levels fall and remain below 250 cells/μL for 1 month, as patients could be susceptible to opportunistic infections [48,56].

Finally, while alefacept is an immune-modulating medication, to date, there have been no clinically significant increased rates of infection or malignancy [8,56].

Summary

The biologic agents are effective drugs to treat psoriasis. They provide physicians with additional options for patients who cannot tolerate traditional therapies or for whom traditional therapies are not sufficient. While these new TNF-α inhibitors and anti–T-cell agents have potential complications, with proper monitoring, they are generally safe. Both physicians and patients should be aware of the risks involved with each medicine so that the correct drug is chosen to suit each patient.

References

[1] Hoekstra M, van Ede AE, Haagsma CJ, et al. Factors associated with toxicity, final dose, and efficacy of methotrexate in patients with rheumatoid arthritis. Ann Rheum Dis 2003;62(5):423–6.

[2] Duhra P. Treatment of gastrointestinal symptoms associated with methotrexate therapy for psoriasis. J Am Acad Dermatol 1993;28(3):466–9.

[3] Lowe NJ, Wieder JM, Rosenbach A, et al. Long-term low-dose cyclosporine therapy for severe psoriasis: effects on renal function and structure. J Am Acad Dermatol 1996;35(5 Pt 1):710–9.

[4] Hojo M, Morimoto T, Maluccio M, et al. Cyclosporine induces cancer progression by a cell-autonomous mechanism. Nature 1999;397(6719):530–4.

[5] Gupta AK, Goldfarb MT, Ellis CN, et al. Side-effect profile of acitretin therapy in psoriasis. J Am Acad Dermatol 1989;20(6):1088–93.

[6] Gronhoj Larsen F, Steinkjer B, Jakobsen P, et al. Acitretin is converted to etretinate only during concomitant alcohol intake. Br J Dermatol 2000;143(6):1164–9.

[7] Weinberg JM, Saini R, Tutrone WD. Biological therapy for psoriasis—the first wave: infliximab, etanercept, efalizumab, and alefacept. J Drugs Dermatol 2002;1(3):303–10.

[8] Stern DK, Tripp JM, Ho VC, et al. The use of systemic immune moderators in dermatology: an update. Dermatol Clin 2005;23(2):259–300.

[9] Gottlieb AB. Infliximab for psoriasis. J Am Acad Dermatol 2003;49:S112–7.

[10] Chaudhari U, Romano P, Mulcahy LD, et al. Efficacy and safety of infliximab monotherapy for plaque-type psoriasis: A randomized trial. Lancet 2001;357:1842–7.

[11] Mease PJ, Goffe BS, Metz J, et al. Etanercept in the treatment of psoriatic arthritis and psoriasis: a randomized trial. Lancet 2000;356:385–90.

[12] Goffe B, Cather JC. Etanercept: an overview. J Am Acad Dermatol 2003;49(2 Suppl):S105–11 Review.

[13] Weinblatt ME, Kremer JM, Bankhurst AD. Trial of etanercept, a recombinant tumor necrosis factor receptor: Fc fusion protein, in patients with rheumatoid arthritis receiving methotrexate. N Engl J Med 1999;340:253–9.

[14] Etanercept [package insert]. Thousand Oaks (CA): Immunex Corp.; 2004.

[15] Gottlieb AB, Matheson R, Lowe NJ, et al. Efficacy of Enbrel in patients with psoriasis. J Invest Dermatol 2002;119:234.

[16] Slifman NR, Gershon SK, Lee JH, et al. Listeria monocytogenes infection as a complication of treatment with tumor necrosis factor alpha-neutralizing agents. Arthritis Rheum 2003;48(2):319–24.

[17] Lee JH, Slifman NR, Gershon SK, et al. Life-threatening histoplasmosis complicating immunotherapy with tumor necrosis factor alpha antagonists infliximab and etanercept. Arthritis Rheum 2002;46(10):2565–70.

[18] Wallis RS, Broder M, Wong J, et al. Reactivation of latent granulomatous infections by infliximab. Clin Infect Dis 2005;41(Suppl 3):S194–8.

[19] Kaplan G, Freedman VH. The role of cytokines in the immune response to tuberculosis. Res Immunol 1996;147:565–72.

[20] Saunders BM, Cooper AM. Restraining mycobacteria: the role of granulomas in mycobacterial infections. Immunol Cell Biol 2000;78:334–41.

[21] Mohan VP, Scanga CA, Yu K, et al. Effects of tumor necrosis factor alpaha on host immune response in

the chronic persistent tuberculosis: possible role for limiting pathology. Infect Immun 2001;69:1847–55.

[22] Hamilton CD. Tuberculosis in the cytokine era: what rheumatologists need to know. Arthritis Rheum 2003;48(8):2085–91.

[23] CDC. Guide for primary health care providers: targeted tuberculin testing and treatment of latent tuberculosis infection 2005. Available at: http://www.cdc.gov/nchstp/tb/pubs//LTBI/default.htm. Accessed July 5, 2006.

[24] Calabrese L. The yin and yang of tumor necrosis factor inhibitors. Cleve Clin J Med 2006;73(3):251–6.

[25] Keane J. TNF-blocking agents and tuberculosis: new drugs illuminate an old topic. Rheumatology (Oxford) 2005;44:714–20.

[26] Kinlen L. Immunosuppressive therapy and acquired immunological disorders. Cancer Res 1992;52(19 Suppl):5474s–6s.

[27] Thomas E, Brewster DH, Black RJ, et al. Risk of malignancy among patients with rheumatic conditions. Int J Cancer 2000;88(3):497–502.

[28] Bernstein CN, Blanchard JF, Kliewer E, et al. Cancer risk in patients with inflammatory bowel disease: a population-based study. Cancer 2001;91(4):854–62.

[29] Hochberg MC, Lebwohl M, Plevy SE, et al. The benefit/risk profile of TNF-blocking agents: findings of a consensus panel. Semin Arthritis Rheum 2005; 34(6):819–36.

[30] Brown SL, Greene MH, Gershon SK, et al. Tumor necrosis factor antagonist therapy and lymphoma development: twenty-six cases reported to the Food and Drug Administration. Arthritis Rheum 2002;46(12):3151–8.

[31] Robinson WH, Genovese MC, Moreland LW. Demyelinating and neurologic events reported in association with tumor necrosis factor alpha antagonism: by what mechanisms could tumor necrosis factor alpha antagonists improve rheumatoid arthritis but exacerbate multiple sclerosis? Arthritis Rheum 2001;44(9):1977–83.

[32] Sicotte NL, Voskuhl RR. Onset of multiple sclerosis associated with anti-TNF therapy. Neurology 2001; 57(10):1885–8.

[33] Mohan N, Edwards ET, Cupps TR, et al. Demyelination occurring during anti-tumor necrosis factor alpha therapy for inflammatory arthritides. Arthritis Rheum 2001;44(12):2862–9.

[34] Anker SD, Coats AJ. How to recover from Renaissance? The significance of the results of Recover, Renaissance, Renewal and Attach. Int J Cardiol 2002; 86(2–3):123–30.

[35] Mann DL, McMurray JJ, Packer M, et al. Targeted anticytokine therapy in patients with chronic heart failure: results of the Randomized Etanercept Worldwide Evaluation (RENEWAL). Circulation 2004;109:1594–602.

[36] Wolfe F, Michaud K. Heart failure in rheumatoid arthritis: rates, predictors, and the effect of anti-tumor necrosis factor therapy. Am J Med 2004; 116:305–11.

[37] Bozkurt B, Torre-Amione G, Warren MS, et al. Results of targeted anti-tumor necrosis factor therapy with etanercept (enbrel) in patients with advanced heart failure. Circulation 2001;103:1044–7.

[38] Infliximab [package insert]. Malvern (PA): Centocor, Inc.; 2005.

[39] Bongartz T, Sutton AJ, Sweeting MJ, et al. Anti-TNF antibody therapy in rheumatoid arthritis and the risk of serious infections and malignancies: systematic review and meta-analysis of rare harmful effects in randomized trials. JAMA 2006;295(19): 2275–85.

[40] Bresnihan B, Cunnane G. Infection complications associated with the use of biologic agents. Rheum Dis Clin North Am 2003;29:185–202.

[41] Keane J, Gershon S, Wise RP, et al. Tuberculosis associated with infliximab, a tumor necrosis factor alpha-neutralizing agent. N Engl J Med 2001;345: 1098–104.

[42] Levine B, Kalman J, Mayer L, et al. Elevated circulating levels of tumor necrosis factor in severe chronic heart failure. N Engl J Med 1990;323: 236–41.

[43] Adalimumab [package insert]. Chicago (IL): Abbott Laboratories; 2005.

[44] Furst DE, Schiff MH, Fleischmann RM, et al. Adalimumab, a fully human anti tumor necrosis factor-alpha monoclonal antibody, and concomitant standard anti-rheumatic therapy for the treatment of rheumatoid arthritis: results of STAR (Safety Trial of Adalimumab in Rheumatoid Arthritis). J Rheumatol 2003;30:2563–71.

[45] Krueger JG. The immunologic basis for the treatment of psoriasis with new biologic agents. J Am Acad Dermatol 2002;46(1):1–23.

[46] Krueger J, Gottlieb A, Miller B, et al. Anti-CD11a treatment for psoriasis concurrently increases circulating T-cells and decreases plaque T-cells, consistent with inhibition of cutaneous T-cell trafficking. J Invest Dermatol 2000;115:333.

[47] Cather JC, Cather JC, Menter A. Modulating T cell responses for the treatment of psoriasis: a focus on efalizumab. Expert Opin Biol Ther 2003;3(2): 361–70.

[48] Weinberg JM. An overview of Infliximab, Etanercept, Efalizumab, and Alefacept as biologic therapy for Psoriasis. Clin Ther 2003;25:1–19.

[49] Efalizumab [package insert]. San Francisco (CA): Genentech, Inc.; 2005.

[50] Leonardi CL. Efalizumab in the treatment of psoriasis. Dermatol Ther 2004;17(5):393–400.

[51] Gaylor ML, Duvic M. Generalized pustular psoriasis following withdrawal of efalizumab. J Drugs Dermatol 2004;3(1):77–9.

[52] Pietrzak A, Chodorowska G, Bartkowiak-Emeryk M, et al. Possibilities of using alefacept in the

treatment of psoriasis. Ann Univ Mariae Curie Sklo-
dowska 2003;58:311-3.

[53] Nickoloff BJ. Characterization of lymphocyte-dependent angiogenesis using a SCID mouse: human skin model of psoriasis. J Investig Dermatol Symp Proc 2000;5:67-73.

[54] Gade JN. Clinical update on alefacept: consideration for use in patients with psoriasis. J Manag Care Pharm 2004;10(3 Suppl B):S33-7.

[55] Gordon KB, Langley RG. Remittive effects of intramuscular alefacept in psoriasis. J Drugs Dermatol 2003;2(6):624-8.

[56] Alefacept [package insert]. Cambridge (MA): Biogen IDEC Inc.; 2005.

[57] Lebwohl M, Enno C, Langley R. An international, randomized, double-blind, placebo-controlled phase 3 trial of intramuscular alefacept in patients with chronic plaque psoriasis. Arch Dermatol 2003;139:719-27.

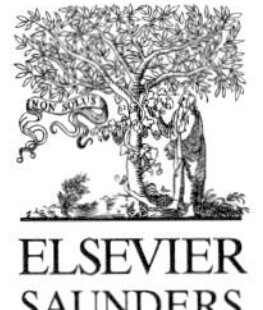

DERMATOLOGIC
CLINICS

Dermatol Clin 25 (2007) 215–221

Drug Reactions Affecting the Nail Unit: Diagnosis and Management

Bianca Maria Piraccini, MD, PhD*, Matilde Iorizzo, MD

Department of Dermatology, University of Bologna, Via Massarenti, 1, Bologna 40138, Italy

Nail abnormalities are an uncommon side effect of drug administration. Although many nail disorders have been associated with drug intake, the great majority of such associations are anecdotal. Most nail changes due to drugs are the outcome of acute toxicity to the nail epithelia and they may involve several or all nails. Nail symptoms vary depending on which nail structure is affected [1–5]. In most cases, nail abnormalities are asymptomatic, but sometimes cause pain and impair manual activities. Several factors may complicate the diagnosis:

Because of the kinetics of nail formation and slow growth rate, the nail changes may appear several weeks after drug intake. This may make it difficult to correlate the abnormalities with the drug.

Nail symptoms often improve or resolve without drug withdrawal.

Rechallenge is often negative.

The abnormalities do not necessarily involve all nails.

Often, the pathogenesis of nail damage is not completely understood.

Teratogenesis

Some drugs, if taken during pregnancy, may interfere with nail development of the fetus. This interference becomes evident in nail abnormalities of newborns. These abnormalities range from mild hypoplasia to complete absence of the nail

(Fig. 1). Distal digit malformation may be associated. Nail hypoplasia may partially improve during the first months of life. Anticonvulsants (eg, carbamazepine, hydantoin, trimethadione, valproic acid) and anticoagulants (eg, warfarin) are the most common drugs producing similar malformations [6,7].

Nail matrix damage

Beau's lines and onychomadesis

Beau's lines and onychomadesis are typical signs of acute and severe toxicity to the nail matrix keratinization with transient decrease or arrest in the nail plate production. The nail plate shows transverse depressions of the surface (Beau's lines) or a whole thickness sulcus that splits the nail plate into two parts (onychomadesis). In Beau's lines, the depth of the depression represents the extent of damage, the width, or the duration of the insult. Onychomadesis is the extreme expression of Beau's lines.

A drug should always be suspected when these signs affect all nails at the same distance from the proximal nail fold. A drug intake of 2 to 3 weeks before the appearance of the nail symptom should be considered, as a fingernail takes about 40 days to emerge from the proximal nail fold. A toenail takes about 80 days to emerge from the proximal nail fold.

Therapies most frequently responsible include cancer chemotherapeutic agents (taxanes) [8], retinoids [9], and radiation therapy. These presentations have also been described with the intake of carbamazepine, cefaloridine and cloxacillin [10], dapsone, fluorine, itraconazole [11], lithium,

* Corresponding author.
E-mail address: bmpiracc@med.unibo.it
(B.M. Piraccini).

0733-8635/07/$ - see front matter © 2007 Elsevier Inc. All rights reserved.
doi:10.1016/j.det.2007.01.006

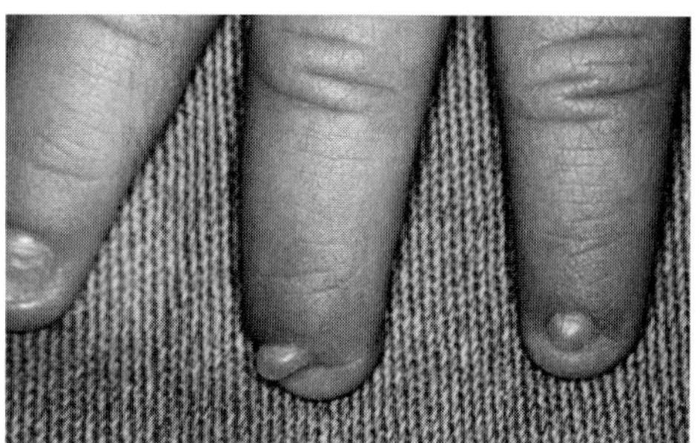

Fig. 1. Micronychia of an infant's second and third fingernails due to anticonvulsants taken by the mother during pregnancy.

metoprolol, phenophtaleine, psoralens, sulfonamides, and tetracyclines.

Drug-induced Beau's lines and onychomadesis are usually dose-related and reproducible with repetitive cycles of drug intake. There is no preventive measure and they require no treatment because they migrate distally as the nail grows.

These nail abnormalities are not exclusive to drug intake, but are also commonly seen after trauma or systemic illness.

Nail fragility

Nail fragility may be a consequence of factors that alter nail plate production (generally a mild damage to the nail matrix) or factors that damage the already keratinized nail plate. Nail plate thinning due to proximal nail matrix damage always involves the whole nail length and is often associated with abnormalities in the superficial nail plate. Damage to the distal nail matrix may produce alterations in the shape of the nail plate free edge, but not of the superficial nail plate.

Clinically we can distinguish two different types of nail fragility:

- Lamellar onychoschizia: The superficial layers of the nail plate show a lamellar exfoliation that starts proximally and may involve the whole nail plate.
- Onychorrhexis: Isolated split at the free edge, which sometimes extends proximally. The nail plate is thin and presents parallel furrows running in the superficial layer.

Nail brittleness is observed in patients treated with cancer chemotherapeutic agents. Retinoids (eg, acitretin, etretinate, and isotretinoin) or antiretroviral agents can be responsible for lamellar onychoschizia.

Nail growth rate alteration

Drugs can decrease or increase nail growth rate. Decreased nail growth can be explained by a reduced mitotic activity of the nail matrix keratinocytes. The mechanism of increased nail growth is not completely understood.

Drugs that have occasionally been reported to induce a decreased nail growth are cyclosporin A, heparin, lithium, methotrexate, and zidovudine. Increased nail growth has been observed in patients treated with fluconazole, itraconazole [12], levodopa [13], and oral contraceptives. Retinoids have been associated with both decreased and increased nail growth.

True transverse leukonychia

True transverse leukonychia is a sign of transient impairment of the distal nail matrix keratinocytes, resulting in the persistence of cell nuclei in the nail plate. True leukonychia appears as one or several parallel transverse white and opaque bands affecting all nails at the same level and moving distally with nail growth. The bands are usually 1 or 2 mm wide. This sign has been reported during treatment with chemotherapeutic agents [14,15], especially doxorubicin, cyclophosphamide, and vincristine. Other responsible drugs are cyclosporin, fluorine, penicillamine, pilocarpine, retinoids, corticosteroids, and sulfonamides. Typically, after acute arsenic and thallium poisoning, the nails show bands of transverse leukonychia called Mees' lines, which are distributed along the entire width of the nail plate. Mees' lines are usually solitary but may be multiple.

Nail bed damage

Onycholysis and photo-onycholysis

Onycholysis and photo-onycholysis are nail changes that result from acute toxicity to the nail bed epithelium with loss of the normal adhesion between the nail bed and the nail plate. With onycholysis and photo-onycholysis, the nail plate is detached from the nail bed and appears white. In photo-onycholysis the detachment is caused by a photo-mediated toxic or allergic effect of the drug. Typically the thumbs are spared. Four types of photo-onycholysis can be distinguished, depending on the site of the detachment.

In type 1, 2, and 3, the detachment involves the central-distal portion of the nail bed (lateral margin spared). In type 4, the detachment involves only the central portion of the nail bed and is often accompanied by hemorrhagic bulla. In type 3, a reddish discoloration of the nail bed is associated. Several nails are usually involved; only one or a few digits are affected in type 2 [16].

Onycholysis, often associated with subungual abscess, is frequent in patients treated with taxane chemotherapeutic agents, such as docetaxel and paclitaxel [17,18]. Possible pathogeneses for taxane-induced nail changes include activation of nociceptive C-fibers that cause or enhance neurogenic inflammation by release of neuropeptides or prostaglandins from sympathetic postganglionic terminals. A cyclooxigenase-2 inhibitor may represent a possible treatment if the latter mechanism is involved [19]. Other drugs reported to be associated with this ungual change are methotrexate [20], retinoids, and infliximab [21].

Photo-onycholysis is typical in patients undergoing psoralen–U-VA therapy (Fig. 2). In this case, development of photo-onycholysis can be prevented by topical application of colored nail varnishes. Captopril, chlorpromazine, doxycycline, thiazide diuretics, oral contraceptives, and fluoroquinolones may also be associated with photo-onycholysis.

Onycholysis and photo-onycholysis often regress spontaneously, even without interrupting drug intake. In some cases they may persist after the drug withdrawal. Rechallenge is usually negative. Soaking the affected digits in topical antiseptic solutions helps prevent microbial colonization.

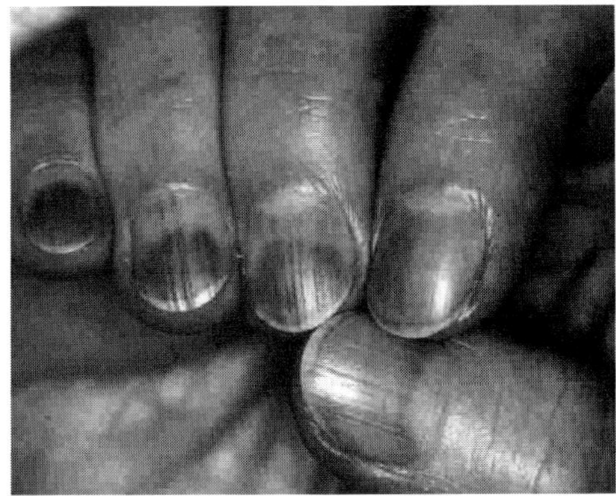

Fig. 2. Photo-onycholysis in a woman undergoing psoralen–U-VA therapy.

Apparent leukonychia

Apparent leukonychia appears as a white pigmentation of the nail plate resulting from nail bed damage. It can be easily distinguished from true leukonychia because it fades with digital compression. Apparent leukonychia appears as transverse parallel pale white bands (Muehrcke's lines) that do not migrate with nail growth. The pathogenesis is unknown. These bands are asymptomatic and are a common side effect of cancer chemotherapy. Apparent leukonychia resolves after drug withdrawal.

Proximal nail fold damage

Acute paronychia

In drug-induced acute paronychia, the proximal nail fold appears erythematous, inflamed, and painful, and several nails are usually involved soon after drug intake.

Loss of the nail plate can be associated with acute paronychia. The pathogenesis is unclear, but a toxic effect of the drug on nail epithelia or a pyogenic infection may be responsible for the clinical presentation.

Exudative severe paronychia may be observed in patients taking methotrexate [22]. Paronychia due to antiretrovirals [23,24] and retinoids [25] is also common (more frequent with isotretinoin) and usually improves as the dosage of the drug is reduced.

Topical steroids and mupirocine can be helpful in reducing inflammation and microbial colonization. Paronychia resolves with drug interruption and is frequently followed by onychomadesis. Rechallenge is often positive.

Pyogenic granulomas

Multiple pyogenic granulomas may arise from proximal and lateral nail folds as a typical side effect of treatment with retinoids (eg, isotretinoin and acitretin) (Fig. 3) and cyclosporin, as well as with the antiretroviral protease-inhibitor indinavir [26,27]. One or several nails show granulation tissue with formation of painful bleeding nodules. The pathogenesis is unknown, but it has been proposed that the drug may activate angiogenic factors. The occurrence of the same side effects with different drugs (eg, retinoids and indinavir) is probably due to the fact that the HIV-1 protease catalytic site and cellular retinoic acid-binding proteins have structural analogies.

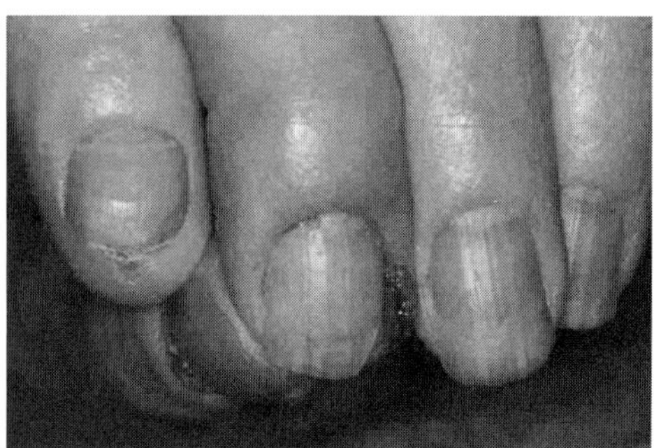

Fig. 3. Pyogenic granulomas arising from proximal and lateral nail folds in a patient taking retinoids.

Paronychia associated with pyogenic granulomas has recently been reported with antiepidermal growth factor receptor antibodies (eg, cetuximab (C225)) [28,29] and epidermal growth factor receptor inhibitors used as chemotherapeutic agents with kinase activity (eg, gefatinib, imatinib, sorafenib, and sunitinib) [30,31]. Nail changes appear from 1 to 3 months after starting treatment. The nail abnormalities fade with interruption of treatment. The reason why some fingers are affected when others are not is unknown.

Topical mupirocin and potent topical corticosteroids may help in relieving the nail symptoms. Topical alitretinoin (9-cis-retinoic acid), a retinoid receptor panagonist, has been suggested as a treatment for pyogenic granuloma [32]. Surgical excision of the granulomas is useless, since relapses are the rule.

Nail blood flow alterations

Ischemic changes

Drugs that impair distal digital perfusion may damage the nail unit with ischemic changes or necrosis. Raynaud's phenomenon is the first typical sign of digital ischemia. When Raynaud's phenomenon occurs, the digit becomes cold and gradually develops gangrene if the blood flow is not restored. These side effects may occur during systemic administration of β-blockers as well as after systemic or intralesional administration of bleomycin.

Noncardioselective β-blockers, especially propanolol, provoke ischemia in response to reduced cardiac output (induced by cardiac β1 blockade). There is no peripheral vasodilation. However, vasoconstriction occurs, induced by peripheral β2 blockade [33].

Bleomycin produces ischemia in a considerable percentage of patients. The side effect usually develops several months after treatment and is due to collagen and glucosaminoglycan deposition with scleroderma-like manifestations [34].

Drug withdrawal is not always associated with regression of the symptoms.

Subungual hemorrhages

Drugs that impair the nail bed blood vessels may damage the nail unit with splinter hemorrhages and subungual hematoma. They are dose-related and slowly disappear after drug withdrawal. Splinter hemorrhages appear as multiple tiny longitudinal streaks that are purple to brown and are most often evident in the distal nail bed. These are almost exclusively seen in the fingernails. The hematoma appears as a red to black discoloration due to trapping of blood at the juncture of the nail plate and nail bed. Hence, these are called subungual hematomas. Over time, a subungual hematoma slowly migrates distally with outgrowth of the nail plate.

Splinter hemorrhages and subungual hematomas are possible side effects of antithrombotics and anticoagulants, including aspirin and warfarin [35]. Cancer chemotherapeutic agents, especially the taxanes [36], and tetracyclines can also cause subungual hemorrhages and hematomas due to thrombocytopenia or extravasation of blood. Recently the authors described a case of splinter hemorrhages due to the nucleotide analog ganciclovir [37].

Nail atrophy

Prolonged application of high-potency topical corticosteroids may produce digital atrophy with bone resorption. In such cases, the affected digit shows a sharpened appearance, thinning, erythema, and scaling of the periungual skin [38].

Nail pigmentation

Melanonychia

Several drugs may activate clusters of nail matrix melanocytes to produce melanin, giving rise to the appearance of a band of melanonychia, or multiple longitudinal or transverse bands ranging in color from light brown to black [39]. In drug-induced melanonychia, several nails are

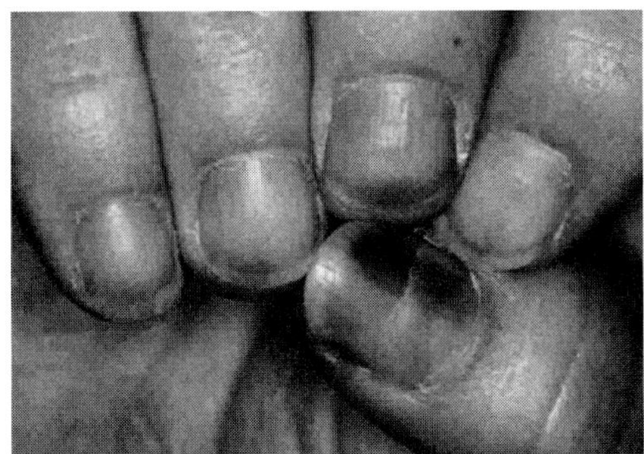

Fig. 4. Longitudinal melanonychia due to radiation therapy.

generally affected with multiple bands. In some cases only one digit is involved.

When the band is isolated, it is important to distinguish a band of longitudinal melanonychia due to drugs from a band of longitudinal melanonychia due to a nail matrix melanocytic neoplasm. In doubtful cases, a nail matrix biopsy is mandatory.

A diffuse activation of nail matrix melanocytes produces pigmentation of the whole nail plate. Drug-induced melanonychia most commonly appears 3 to 8 weeks after drug intake. Pigmentation is usually reversible within 6 to 8 weeks, but may persist for months after drug interruption. Rechallenge is usually negative. The pathogenesis of nail melanocyte activation is unclear and is independent of melanocyte-stimulating hormone and corticotropin activity and ultraviolet light.

Drugs responsible for melanonychia include zidovudine, cancer chemotherapeutic agents [40], hydroxyurea [41] and psoralens [42]. Radiation therapy for malignant disease far from the digit can also cause longitudinal melanonychia [43] (Fig. 4).

Nonmelanic pigmentation

Nail pigmentation may be a consequence of storage within the nail plate by systemic drugs that are excreted via the nail unit. The pigmentation typically moves distally with nail growth. Tetracyclines [44] and gold salts [45] often produce a yellow discoloration of the nail plate. Clofazimine produces a dark-brown pigmentation [46].

In other cases, nail pigmentation may be a consequence of dermal deposition by systemic drugs. Pigmentation of the periungual tissues may be associated. The pigmentation does not move as the nail grows. It takes several months to decrease after interruption of therapy and may not disappear completely.

Minocycline may cause a blue-gray pigmentation [47] of the nail bed, although this is rare, and antimalarials may produce a blue-brown pigmentation [48].

Several topical drugs, such as tar and anthralin, may deposit within the superficial layers of the nail plate, producing an exogenous brown-black pigmentation. Exogenous pigmentation migrates distally with nail growth and has a proximal border parallel to the cuticle.

Summary

An accurate clinical history is essential to diagnose drug-induced nail changes. Drug-induced nail alteration should be suspected when several or all nails are affected. The drugs that most commonly cause nail abnormalities are cancer chemotherapeutic agents, systemic retinoids, and indinavir. Only a few classes of drugs produce reproducible nail changes in a significant number of patients.

How cancer chemotherapeutic agents could have such pleotropic effects on the different parts of the nail unit is unknown.

Most of these changes are a consequence of direct toxicity to the nail epithelia, but other possible mechanism may be involved. Drug-induced nail abnormalities are often not related to drug dosage and sometimes might persist after drug interruption.

The study of drug-induced nail changes may offer new insights into further knowledge of nail physiology and of mechanisms of action of some drugs.

References

[1] Tosti A, Baran R, Dawber RPR. The nail in systemic diseases and drug-induced changes. In: Baran R, Dawber RPR, de Berker DAR, et al, editors. Baran and Dawber's diseases of the nails and their management. 2nd edition. Oxford: Blackwell Science; 2001. p. 223–9.

[2] Daniel CR III, Scher RK. Nail changes secondary to systemic drugs or ingestans. J Am Acad Dermatol 1984;10:250–8.

[3] Piraccini BM, Tosti A. Drug-induced nail disorders. Incidence, management and prognosis. Drug Saf 1999;21:187–201.

[4] Piraccini BM, Iorizzo M, Tosti A. Drug-induced nail abnormalities. Am J Clin Dermatol 2003;4:31–7.

[5] Piraccini BM, Iorizzo M, Antonucci A, et al. Drug-induced nail abnormalities. Expert Opin Drug Saf 2004;3:57–65.

[6] Pettifor JM, Benson R. Congenital malformation with the administration of oral anticoagulant during pregnancy. J Pediatr 1975;86:459–62.

[7] Holmes LB, Harvey EA, Brown KS, et al. Anti-convulsant teratogenesis: I. A study design for newborn infants. Teratology 1994;49:202–7.

[8] Minisini AM, Tosti A, Sobrero AF, et al. Taxane-induced nail changes: incidence, clinical presentation and outcome. Ann Oncol 2003;14:333–7.

[9] Baran R. Retinoids and the nail. J Dermatolog Treat 1990;1:151–4.

[10] Eastwood JB, Curtis JR, Smith EK, et al. Shedding of nails apparently induced by the administration of large amounts of cephaloridine and cloxacillin in two anephric patients. Br J Dermatol 1969;81:750–2.

[11] Chen HH, Liao YH. Beau's lines associated with itraconazole. Acta Derm Venereol 2002;82:398.

[12] de Doncker P, Pierard GE. Acquired nail beading in patients receiving itraconazole—an indicator of faster nail growth? A study using optical profilometry. Clin Exp Dermatol 1994;19:404–6.

[13] Miller E. Levodopa and nail growth. N Engl J Med 1973;288:916.

[14] Chapman S, Cohen PR. Transverse leukonychia in patients receiving cancer chemotherapy. South Med J 1997;90:395–8.

[15] Shelley WB, Humprey GB. Transverse leukonychia (Mees' lines) due to daunorubicin chemotherapy. Pediatr Dermatol 1997;14:144–5.

[16] Baran R, Juhlin L. Photoonycholysis. Photodermatol Photoimmunol Photomed 2002;18:202–7.

[17] Hussain S, Anderson DN, Salvatti ME, et al. Onycholysis as a complication of systemic chemotherapy: report of five cases associated with prolonged weekly paclitaxel therapy and review of the literature. Cancer 2000;88:2367–71.

[18] Vanhooteghem O, Richert B, Vindevoghel A, et al. Subungual abscess: a new ungual side effect related to docetaxel therapy. Br J Dermatol 2000;143:462–4.

[19] Wasner G, Hilpert F, Baron R, et al. Nail changes secondary to docetaxel. Lancet 2001;357:910.

[20] Chang JC. Acute bullous dermatosis and onycholysis due to high-dose methotrexate and leucovorin calcium. Arch Dermatol 1987;123:990–2.

[21] Gaylis N. Infliximab in the treatment of an HIV positive patient with Reiter's syndrome. J Rheumatol 2003;30:407–11.

[22] Wantzin GL, Thomsen K. Acute paronychia after high-dose methotrexate therapy. Arch Dermatol 1983;119:623–4.

[23] Zerboni R, Angius AG, Cusini M, et al. Lamivudine-induced paronychia. Lancet 1998;351:1256.

[24] Tosti A, Piraccini BM, D'Antuono A, et al. Paronychia associated with antiretroviral therapy. Br J Dermatol 1999;140:1165–8.

[25] Blumental G. Paronychia and pyogenic granuloma-like lesions with isotretinoin. J Am Acad Dermatol 1984;10:677–8.

[26] Bouscarat F, Bouchard C, Bouhour D. Paronychia and pyogenic granuloma of the great toes in patients with indinavir. N Engl J Med 1998; 338:1776–7.

[27] Calista D, Boschini A. Cutaneous side effects induced by indinavir. Eur J Dermatol 2000;10: 292–6.

[28] Busam KJ, Capodieci P, Motzer R, et al. Cutaneous side effects in cancer patients treated with the antiepidermal growth factor receptor antibody C225. Br J Dermatol 2001;144:1169–76.

[29] Boucher KW, Davidson K, Mirakhur B, et al. Paronychia induced by cetuximab, an antiepidermal growth factor receptor antibody. J Am Acad Dermatol 2002;47:632–3.

[30] Nakano J, Nakamura M. Paronychia induced by gefitinib, an epidermal growth factor receptor tyrosine kinase inhibitor. J Dermatol 2003;30:261–2.

[31] Robert C, Soria JC, Spatz A, et al. Cutaneous side-effects of kinase inhibitors and blocking antibodies. Lancet Oncol 2005;6:491–500.

[32] Maloney DM, Schmidt JD, Duvic M. Alitretinoin gel to treat pyogenic granuloma. J Am Acad Dermatol 2002;47:969–70.

[33] Stringer MD, Bentley PG. Peripheral gangrene associated with β-blockade. Br J Surg 1986;73:1008.

[34] Snauwaert J, Degreef H. Bleomycin-induced Raynaud's phenomenon and acral sclerosis. Dermatologica 1984;169:172–4.

[35] Varotti C, Ghetti E, Piraccini BM, et al. Subungual hematoma in a patient treated with an oral anticoagulant (warfarin sodium). Eur J Dermatol 1997;7: 395–6.

[36] Ghetti E, Piraccini BM, Tosti A. Onycholysis and subungual haemorrhages secondary to systemic chemotherapy (paclitaxel). J Eur Acad Dermatol Venereol 2003;17:459–60.

[37] Lorenzi S, D'Antuono A, Iorizzo M, et al. Skin rash and splinter haemorrhages from ganciclovir. J Dermatolog Treat 2003;14:177–8.

[38] Wolf R, Tur E, Brenner S. Corticosteroid-induced "disappearing digit". J Am Acad Dermatol 1990; 23:755–6.

[39] Baran R, Kechijian P. Longitudinal melanonychia: diagnosis and management. J Am Acad Dermatol 1989;21:1165–75.

[40] Nixon DW. Alterations in nail pigment with cancer chemotherapy. Arch Intern Med 1976;136:1117–8.

[41] Aste N, Fumo G, Contu F, et al. Nail pigmentation caused by hydroxyurea: report of 9 cases. J Am Acad Dermatol 2002;47:146–7.

[42] Ledbetter LS, Hsu S. Melanonychia associated with PUVA therapy. J Am Acad Dermatol 2003;48:31–2.

[43] Shelley WB, Rawnsley HM, Pillsbury DM. Postirradiation melanonychia. Arch Dermatol 1964;90: 174–6.

[44] Hendricks AA. Yellow lunulae with fluorescence after tetracycline therapy. Arch Dermatol 1980;116: 438–40.

[45] Fam AG, Paton TW. Nail pigmentation after parenteral gold therapy for rheumatoid arthritis: "gold nails". Arthritis Rheum 1984;27:119–20.

[46] Tosti A, Piraccini BM, Guerra L. Reversible melanonychia due to clofazimine. 18th World Congress of Dermatology, New York, (1992): 183A.

[47] Kimyai-Asadi A, Jih MH. Minocycline induced nail-bed pigmentation. J Drugs Dermatol 2002;1: 197–8.

[48] Tuffanelli D, Abraham RK, Dubois EI. Pigmentation from antimalarial therapy. Arch Dermatol 1963; 88:113–20.

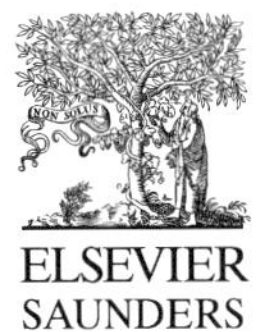

ELSEVIER
SAUNDERS

Dermatol Clin 25 (2007) 223–231

DERMATOLOGIC
CLINICS

Drug Reactions Affecting Hair: Diagnosis

Antonella Tosti, MD*, Massimiliano Pazzaglia, MD

Department of Dermatology, University of Bologna, Via Massarenti 1, 40138 Bologna, Italy

Drugs may cause hair loss, stimulate hair growth or induce changes in the hair shape and color (Table 1). Drug-induced hair loss is, in most cases, a consequence of a toxic effect of the drug on the hair matrix. Although a large number of drugs have been occasionally reported to produce hair loss, the relationship between drug intake and hair loss has been proven only for a few agents (Box 1). Type of hair loss (telogen effluvium, anagen effluvium, or both) depends on the drug, its dosage, and patient's susceptibility. Drug-induced hair loss is usually reversible [1].

Types of drug-induced hair loss

Telogen effluvium

Telogen effluvium is the most common form of hair loss induced by drugs and is characterized by excessive shedding of telogen hairs. Drugs can induce telogen effluvium through three different mechanisms:

1. In most cases, drugs induce telogen effluvium by precipitating the follicle into premature rest.
2. Telogen effluvium may be a consequence of discontinuation of drugs that prolong the duration of anagen such as topical minoxidil and oral contraceptives.
3. Some drugs may cause premature detachment of the club hair from the follicles with shortening of the normal telogen phase (example systemic retinoids).

Hair loss typically occurs about 3 months after beginning of treatment. Patients complain of increased hair shedding, which may be associated with scalp paresthesia or pain (trychodinia). Daily hair shedding is variable, but usually ranges between 100 and 150. Severe hair shedding (more than 200 to 300 hairs daily) is uncommon and is almost exclusively seen with antineoplastic agents, interferons, antiretroviral drugs, and heparin. Hair density may be normal or decreased (Fig. 1). Loss of pubic or body hairs can occasionally occur.

Anagen effluvium

Anagen effluvium is almost exclusively seen after intake of cytotoxic drugs and is usually associated with telogen hair loss.

Hair shedding is usually acute and severe and may produce loss of most of the scalp hair, eyebrows, and eyelashes; other body hairs are less commonly involved (Fig. 2).

Cicatricial alopecia

Diffuse and permanent hair thinning attributable to hair follicle destruction is uncommon and almost exclusively seen after busulphan conditioning for bone marrow transplantation or after radiation therapy for brain tumors.

Reversible hair loss

Anticoagulants

Telogen effluvium is a common side effect of treatment with anticoagulants. It occurs in up to 50% of patients treated with high dosages of heparin, heparinoids, or coumarin derivatives.

Antineoplastic agents

Hair loss is the most common cutaneous side effect of antineoplastic drugs. Hair loss is more frequent and severe in patients receiving combination chemotherapy than in those treated with

---

* Corresponding author.
E-mail address: tosti@med.unibo.it (A. Tosti).

Table 1
Changes in hair color/shape/texture

Hair graying	Hair darkening	Straightening	Curling/kinking
Althesin	Indinavir	Interferon	Antineoplastics
Benzoylperoxide	Antineoplastics (flag-sign)	Lithium	Indinavir
Butyrophenones	Arsenic		Retinoids
Chloroquine	Bromocriptine		Valproic acid
Cyclosporine A (poliosis)	Carbidopa		
Etretinate	Diazoxide		
Hydroquinone	Estrogens		
Interferon-α	Minoxidil		
Mephenesine	Para-aminobenzoic acid		
Phenols	Prostaglandin analogs		
Phenylthiourea	Radiation (electron beam therapy)		
Triparanol	Tamoxifen		
	Verapamil		
	Zidovudine		

monotherapy (Table 2). Severity of hair loss varies among patients submitted to the same therapeutic regimen.

In most patients, hair loss starts after the first or the second cycle of administration of chemotherapy and therefore 4 to 8 weeks after the start of treatment. Evaluation of hair shedding in a group of patients submitted to polychemotherapy with cyclophosphamide, methotrexate, and 5-fluorouracil revealed that mean daily hair shedding was 125 hairs per day but some patients may shed more than 1000 hairs daily [2]. Microscopic examination revealed both telogen and fractured hairs. Other common effects of drug toxicity on hair formation are hair depigmentation and Pohl-Pinkus marks that consist of constrictions of the hair shaft. Hair regrowth is usually very fast after discontinuation of therapy but hair shape and color may be altered.

In rare cases, hair regrowth is not complete and a permanent hair thinning persists.

Antiretroviral drugs

Severe telogen effluvium and patchy hair loss resembling alopecia areata are common side effects of indinavir therapy, occurring in up to 10% of patients. Leg, thigh, pubic, thoracic, and axillary hair are also frequently affected. Combined treatment with indinavir and ritonavir may be associated with severe hair loss since ritonavir increases the plasma concentration of indinavir [3]. The combination of lopinavir plus ritonavir has also been associated with hair loss [4]. Indinavir can also induce hair darkening or cause changes in the hair texture and shape. Hypertrichosis and darkening of the pubic hair has been reported in patients taking zidovudine (AZT).

Oral contraceptives

Interruption of oral contraceptive therapy is frequently followed by telogen effluvium. This is because the estrogens contained in the contraceptives prolong anagen duration and synchronize the hair cycle, which is followed by a transition into telogen of a large number of follicles after estrogen interruption. In some cases, however, transient hair loss is seen 3 to 5 months after beginning of treatment with oral contraceptives [5]. Contraceptives containing androgenic progestational agents (the nortestosterone-derivatives levonorgestrel) may induce or worsen androgenetic alopecia.

Progestin-releasing implants

Acne, androgenetic alopecia, and hirsutism are possible side effects of levonorgestrel-releasing implants because of the androgenic effects of progestational drugs. Side effects are more common in the initial months of use, when the progestin levels are higher than in the later months [6].

Gonadotropine-releasing hormone agonist

Androgenetic alopecia has been reported in children treated with triptorelin for precocious puberty [7]. Goserelin may cause hair loss and androgenetic alopecia in susceptible women [8].

Box 1. Drugs reported to produce hair loss

ACE inhibitors (captopril, enalapril,
  moexipril, ramipril)
Allopurinol
Amiodarone
Amphetamines[a]
Analgesics/antinflammatories (ibuprofen,
  indomethacin, naproxen)
Androgens[a,d]
Anticoagulants (coumarins, dextran,
  heparin/heparinoids)[a]
Antiepileptics (carbamazepine,
  hydantoines, troxidone, valproic acid,
  vigabatrin)[a]
Antipsychotics (flupenthixol decanoate,
  fluphenazine decanoate)
Antithiroid drugs (carbimazole, iodine,
  thiouracil)[a]
Appetite suppressants
Aromatase inhibitors (fadrozole, 4-OHA,
  vorozole)[a,d]
Benzimidazoles (albendazole,
  mebendazole)
β blockers (levobunolol, metoprolol,
  nadolol, propanolol, timolol)[a]
Bromocriptine
Buspiron
214 bis Busulphan[b]
Butyrrophenones
Cantharidine
Cholestyramine
Chloramphenicol
Cidofovir
Cimetidine
Clonazepam
Clotrimazole
Colchicine
Contraceptives (oral)[e]
Danazol
Diclofenac
Dixyrazine
Dyazoxide
Ethambutol
Etionamide
Gentamicin
Glatiramer acetate
Glibenclamide
Gold salts
G-CSF (granulocyte-colony stimulating
  factor)
Haloperidol
Hypocholesterolemic drugs (clofibrate,
  fenofibrate)
Immunoglobulins

Indandiones
Indinavir[a]
Interferons[a]
Isonicotinic acid hydrazide[c]
Leflunomide[a]
Levodopa
Lithium[a]
Maprotilene
Mesalazine
Methyldopa
Methysergide
Methyrapone
Minoxidil[e]
Nicotinic acid
Nitrofurantoin
Octreotide
Olanzapine
Pentosone polysulphate
Phenindione
Piroxicam
Potassium thiocyanate
Pyridostigmine
Radiation (<700 Gy)[a,c]
Retinol (vitamin A)[a]
Retinoids (acitretin, etretinate,
  isotrctinoin)[a]
Risperidone
Salicylates
Serotonin uptake inhibitors
  (fluoxetin, paroxetine)[a]
Spironolactone
Sulphasalazine
Tamoxifene
Terbinafine
Terfenadine
Thiamphenicol
Thrimetadione
Thyroxine
Tocopherol (vitamin E)
Trazodone
Triazoles (fluconazole, itraconazole)
Tricyclic antidepressants (amytriptiline
  desipramine, doxepin, imipramine,
  maprotiline)
Triparanol
Vasopressin

---

[a] Established by multiple reports or proved
by rechallange.
[b] May produce permanent alopecia.
[c] May produce anagen effluvium.
[d] May produce androgenetic alopecia.
[e] May produce telogen effluvium 3 months
after discontinuation.

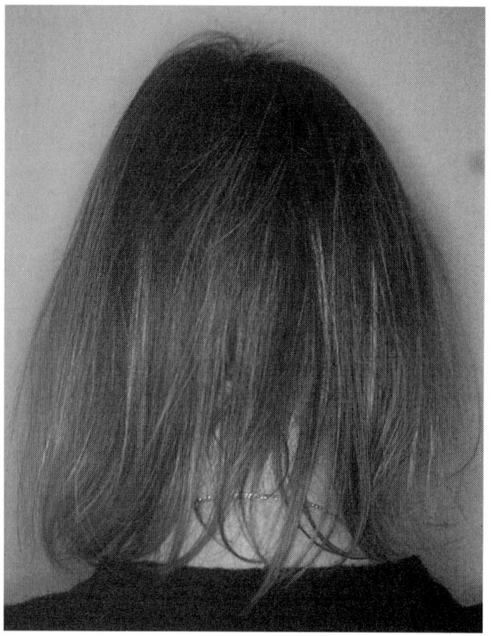

Fig. 1. Telogen effluvium attributable to heparin: the patient complains of reduced hair density after severe shedding.

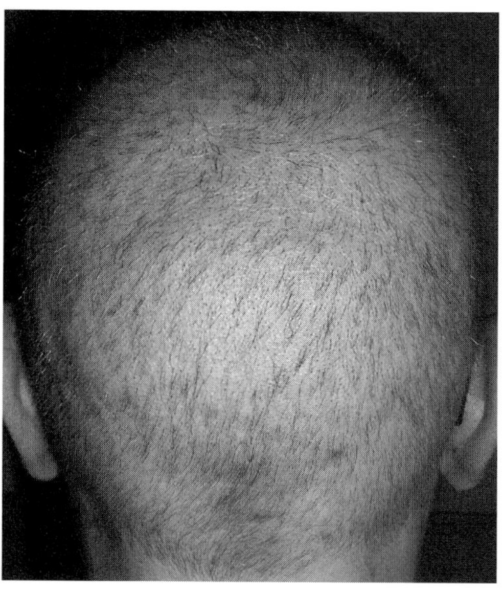

Fig. 2. Severe alopecia in a patient undergoing combination chemotherapy.

Antiestrogens and aromatase inhibitors

Tamoxifen and nonsteroidal aromatase inhibitors are widely used for the therapy of hormone-sensitive breast cancer.

Tamoxifen has been occasionally associated with hair thinning and discoloration. Androgenetic alopecia is one of the most common side effects of treatment with the nonsteroidal aromatase inhibitors letrozole and vorozole [9].

Esterified estrogens–methyltestosterone replacement therapy

Up to 12% of women receiving oral esterified estrogens–methyltestosterone combinations for the treatment of menopause experience alopecia and/or other androgen-dependent skin signs such as acne and hirsutism [10].

Table 2
Risk of hair loss with different chemotherapy drugs

Drugs that usually do cause hair loss	Drugs that sometimes cause hair loss	Drugs that usually don't cause hair loss
Adriamycin	Amsacrine	Capecitabine
Cyclophosphamide	Bleomycin	Carmustine
Daunorubicin	Busulphan	Carboplatin
Docetaxel	Cytarabine	Cisplatin
Epirubicin	5-Fluorouracil	Fludarabine
Etoposide	Gemcitabine	6-Mercaptopurine
Ifosfamide	Lomustine	Procarbazine
Irinotecan	Melphalan	Raltitrexed
Paclitaxel	Methotrexate-	
Topotecan	Mitoxantrone	
Vindesine	Mitomycin C	
Vinorelbine	Thiotepa	
	Vincristine	
	Vinblastine	

Extracorporeal membrane oxygenation

This techique is used for cardiopulmonary support in a variety of clinical situations. Hair loss after extracorporeal membrane oxygenation is common, occurring in up to 87% of patients [11].

Immunosuppressive drugs

Alopecia is a frequent complication of oral tacrolimus therapy following transplantation, occurring in 28% of cases [12].

Mycophenolate mofetil has also been associated with alopecia. Alopecia occurs in 10% to 16% of patients taking leflunomide, a novel immunomodulatory agent used for the treatment of rheumatoid arthritis [13].

Interferons

Hair loss occurs in up to 50% of patients and is not dose-related. Hair shedding is reversible after interruption of treatment and in some cases despite continuation of therapy [14]. Transient localized alopecia can also occur at the site of interferon-alpha (IFN-α) injections.

Changes in hair shape and color have also been reported subsequent to interferon use. Hair whitening was observed in 18% of patients treated with a low dose of IFN-α for malignant melanoma [15]. Acquired hair straightening has been reported in patients treated with IFN-α plus ribavirin for hepatitis B virus infection. Symptoms regressed after drug discontinuation and recurred after drug reintroduction.

Minoxidil

Telogen effluvium occurs 2 to 3 months after topical minoxidil interruption. Hair loss is often severe and results from simultaneous telogen entry of all follicles that had prolonged their growth under minoxidil stimulation.

Treatment with finasteride 1 mg daily does not prevent telogen effluvium in patients who discontinue topical minoxidil [16].

Hair loss occurring at the beginning of minoxidil therapy is because minoxidil stimulates resting follicles to reenter anagen and therefore induces detachment of the old club hair.

Psychotropic drugs

We are often faced with patients taking psychotropic drugs for the psychological distress caused by hair loss who inquire about possible negative effects of these drugs on hair growth. Although it may be difficult to give a definitive answer to this question, we have summarized here the most relevant information on this topic, keeping in mind that data about frequency of hair loss are not available for most drugs [17,18].

Mood stabilizers

Lithium causes hair loss in up to 20% of long-term users, which may be a consequence of lithium-induced hypothyroidism. Hair straightening has also been associated with lithium intake. Valproic acid and divalproex frequently cause dose-dependent hair loss that may affect up to 12% of patients. Carbamazepine on the other hand is only very rarely responsible for hair loss.

Dopaminergic therapy

Reversible telogen effluvium has been documented in patients with Parkinson's disease treated with dopaminergic drugs including levodopa and both ergot alkaloid and non–ergot alkaloid dopamine receptor agonists (bromocriptine, pramipexole, ropinirole, pergolide, cabergoline). Hair loss is more common in female patients. The mechanism of hair loss during dopoaminergic treatment is still unclear.

Antidepressants

Telogen effluvium has been mainly reported in patients taking the serotonin reuptake inhibitor fluoxetine. It usually occurs a few months after the beginning of therapy but can occasionally develop even more than 1 year after the beginning of treatment. Hair loss has been occasionally reported with tricyclic antidepressants but not with monoamine oxidase inhibitors.

Anxiolytics

Barbiturates and benzodiazepines have not been associated with hair loss.

Fluoroscopy

Temporary patchy alopecia is a possible side effect of neurosurgical operations with prolonged fluoroscopic imaging. Hair loss usually involves the retroauricular areas that receive the highest doses during fluoroscopy and may closely resemble alopecia areata [19].

Retinol (vitamin A)/retinoids

High dosages of vitamin A have been associated with hair loss. In our experience mild hair loss is frequent in patients taking vitamin supplements containing vitamin A. Concurrent administration of vitamin E may potentiate vitamin A toxicity.

Acitretin and isotretinoin cause hair loss with visible alopecia in a high percentage of patients. The side effect is dose-related and may also affect body hair. In some cases alopecia may be severe and total alopecia has also been reported. Premature teloptosis probably has an important role in retinoid-induced hair loss.

Hair lightening and acquired hair kinking are other possible side effects of retinoids (Fig. 3).

Permanent alopecia

Busulphan

Busulphan conditioning for allogeneic or autologous bone marrow transplantation produces permanent alopecia in up to 50% of patients (Fig. 4) [20].

Radiation

Radiotherapy of brain tumors often produces cicatricial alopecia. X-ray dosages higher than 700 Gy in fact permanently destroy the hair follicle. The irradiated area is not completely bald as the follicles that were in telogen at the time of radiation can survive the toxic damage (Fig. 5).

Lichen planopilaris

Lichen planopilaris can be precipitated by antihypertensive agents such angiotensin-converting enzyme (ACE) inhibitors and β-receptor blocking agents. Drug-induced lichen planopilaris is usually rapidly progressive and unresponsive to systemic corticosteroid treatment. It is advisable to substitute these agents with other antihypertensive drugs in patients with active lichen planopilaris.

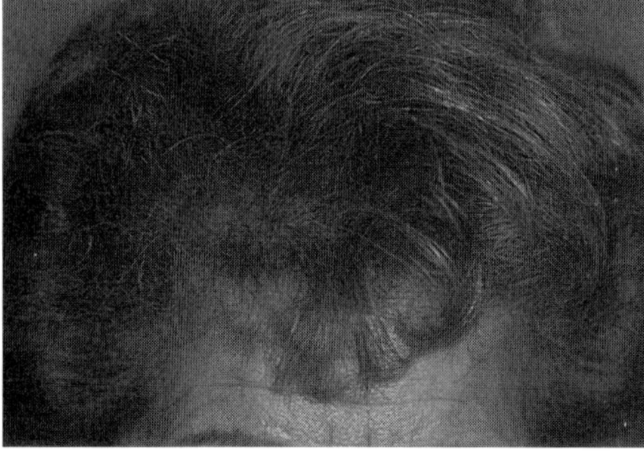

Fig. 3. Hair thinning and kinking during acitretin treatment.

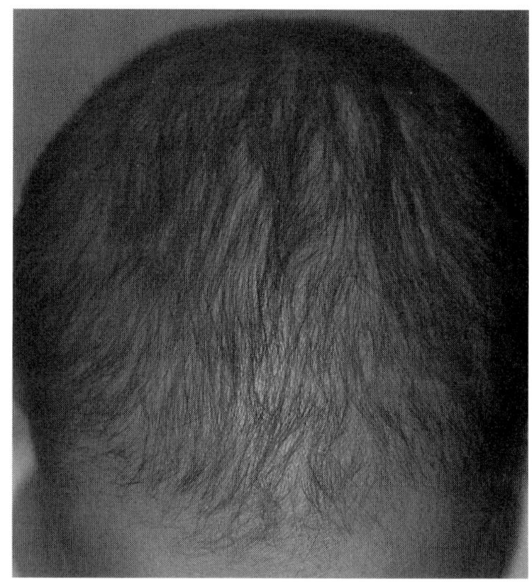

Fig. 4. Cicatricial alopecia attributable to busulphan. The patient experienced diffuse hair thinning after bone marrow transplantation. The pathology showed reduced hair density.

Excessive hair growth

Hirsutism may be a consequence of drugs with androgenic effect and is associated with other signs of hyperandrogenism such as acne, seborrhea, and androgenetic alopecia. Hypertrichosis is a possible side effect of several drugs that stimulate hair growth (Table 3).

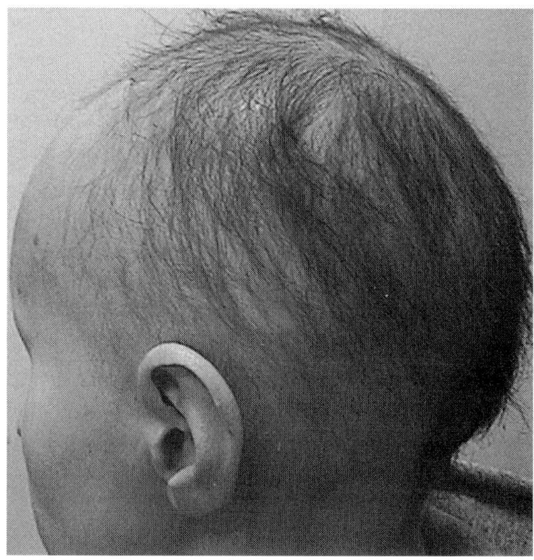

Fig. 5. Cicatricial alopecia after radiotherapy for a brain tumor.

Table 3
Drugs reported to produce hirsutism/hypertrichosis

Hirsutism	Hypertrichosis
ACTH	Acetazolamide
Anabolizing steroids	Albendazole
Androgens	Benoxaprofen
Carbamazepine	Beta blockers (atenolol, betaxolol)
Danazol	Calcium antagonists (niphedipin, verapamil)
Methyrapone	Cetuximab
	Colestiramine
	Copper
	Cyclosporin A[a]
	Desipramine
	Diazoxide
	Diltiazem
	Erythropoietin
	Etambutole
	Etionamide
	Fenoterol
	Gentamycin
	Hexachlorobenzene
	Hydantoins[a]
	Immunoglobulins
	Indometacin
	Interferons
	Melphalan
	Mercury
	Metotrexate
	Methyldopa
	Methyrapone
	Minoxidil
	Mitomycin
	Mitoxantrone
	Nitrosureas
	Penicillamine
	Phenothiazines
	Photochemotherapy
	Pinacidil
	Procarbazine
	Prostaglandin analogs
	Psoralens
	Radiotherapy
	Retinoic acid (tretinoin)
	Sodium tetradecyl sulfate
	Steroids (systemic/topical)
	Streptomycin
	Tacrolimus[a]
	Temposide
	Thallium
	Thiotepa
	Triciclic antidepressants (imipramine, maprotiline)
	Vasoprexine
	Vinblastine
	Vincristine
	Zidovudine

[a] Also cause gingival hyperplasia.

Cyclosporin A

Reversible hypertrichosis is common and most frequently affects the face, back, and eyelashes. It is dose-related, occurring in up to 50% of patients taking high dosages of the drugs after transplantation. It is rarely seen (3% of patients) with dosages less than 5 mg/kg per day (Fig. 6).

Prostaglandin analogs

Eyedrops containing the prostaglandin F analogs (latanoprost, bimatoprost, and travoprost) used for the topical treatment of glaucoma can induce trichomegaly and darkening of the eyelashes [21].

Minoxidil

Hypertrichosis is a common side effect of topical minoxidil and normally involves the face and neck because of inadvertent topical transfer of the drug to anatomic sites other than the scalp (Fig. 7). Hypertrichosis is more common in women. Some women using 5% topical minoxidil develop diffuse hypertrichosis that is probably a result of systemic absorption [22].

Diagnosis and management

Diagnosis

- Consider all drugs taken until 4 months before the onset of hair loss.
- The causative role of the drug is often difficult to prove; normalization of hair loss may, in fact, require 2 to 3 months after drug discontinuation.

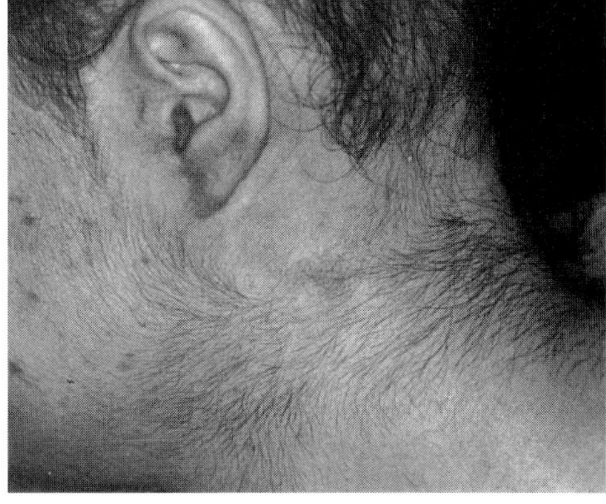

Fig. 6. Severe hypertrichosis in a patient taking cyclosporin (3 mg/kg/day) for alopecia areata.

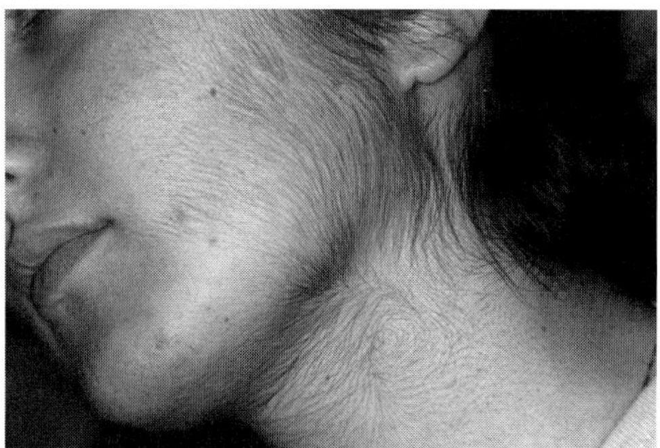

Fig. 7. Severe hypertrichosis in a patient treated with 5% topical minoxidil.

- Perform a pull test and examine the hair under the microscope to determine type of alopecia.

Management

Telogen effluvium

Although telogen effluvium usually resolves spontaneously, it may precipitate or aggravate androgenetic alopecia in predisposed individuals. Discontinuing the causative drug may not improve hair thinning and treatment with finasteride or topical minoxidil may be necessary.

Anagen effluvium

Anticancer-induced hair loss often has a severe negative impact on the patient's quality of life. Available options include scalp hypothermia and topical minoxidil.

Scalp hypothermia represents the only available preventive measure. The efficacy of scalp cooling depends on the cytostatic regimen [23]. In particular, scalp cooling is effective when anthracyclines or taxanes are used alone but not in combination. There are two scientific rationales for scalp cooling. The first is vasoconstriction, which reduces the blood flow to the hair follicles during peak plasma concentrations of the chemotherapeutic agents and so reduces cellular uptake of these agents. The second rationale is reduced biochemical activity, which makes hair follicles less susceptible to the damage of chemotherapeutic agents.

Topical minoxidil has been shown to accelerate hair regrowth after chemotherapy but not prevent hair loss [24].

References

[1] Tosti A, Misciali C, Piraccini BM, et al. Drug-induced hair-loss and hair growth. Drug Saf 1994;10: 310–7.

[2] Bleiker TO, Nicolaou N, Traulsen J, et al. Atrophic telogen effluvium from cytotoxic drugs and a randomized controlled trial to investigate the possible protective effect of pretreatment with a topical vitamin D analogue in humans. Br J Dermatol 2005;153: 103–12.

[3] Ginarte M, Losada E, Prieto A, et al. Generalized hair loss induced by indinavir plus ritonavir therapy. AIDS 2002;16(16):1695–6.

[4] Bongiovanni M, Chiesa E, Monforte A, et al. Hair loss in an HIV-1 infected woman receiving lopinavir plus ritonavir therapy as first line HAART. Dermatol Online J 2003;9:28.

[5] Hair loss and contraceptives. Br Med J 1973;2(5865): 499–500.

[6] Brache V, Faundes A, Alvarez F, et al. Nonmenstrual adverse events during use of implantable contraceptives for women: data from clinical trials. Contraception 2002;65:63–74.

[7] Kauschansky A, Lurie R, Ingber A. Hair loss in children on long-acting gonadotropin-releasing hormone agonist triptorelin treatment. Acta Derm Venereol 1997;77:333.

[8] Gateley CA, Bundred NJ. Alopecia and breast disease. BMJ 1997;314(7079):481.

[9] Simpson D, Curran MP, Perry CM. Letrozole: a review of its use in postmenopausal women with breast cancer. Drugs 2004;64:1213–30.

[10] Phillips E, Bauman C. Safety surveillance of esterified estrogens-methyltestosterone (Estratest and Estratest HS) replacement therapy in the United States. Clin Ther 1997;19:1070–84.

[11] Pettignano R, Heard ML, Labuz MD, et al. Hair loss after extracorporeal membrane oxygenation. Pediatr Crit Care Med 2003;4:363–6.

[12] Tricot L, Lebbe C, Pillebout E, et al. Tacrolimus-induced alopecia in female kidney-pancreas transplant recipients. Transplantation 2005;15(80):1546–9.

[13] Smolen JS, Emery P. Efficacy and safety of leflunomide in active rheumatoid arthritis. Rheumatology (Oxford) 2000;39(Suppl 1):48–56.

[14] Tosti A, Misciali C, Bardazzi F, et al. Telogen effluvium due to recombinant interferon alpha-2b. Dermatology 1992;184:124–5.

[15] Guillot B, Blazquez L, Bessis D, et al. A prospective study of cutaneous adverse events induced by low-dose alpha-interferon treatment for malignant melanoma. Dermatology 2004;208:49–54.

[16] Tosti A, Iorizzo M, Vincenzi C. Finasteride treatment may not prevent telogen effluvium after minoxidil withdrawal. Arch Dermatol 2003;139: 1221–2.

[17] Gautam M. Alopecia due to psychotropic medications. Ann Pharmacother 1999;33:631–7.

[18] Mercke Y, Sheng H, Khan T, et al. Hair loss in psychopharmacology. Ann Clin Psychiatry 2000;12: 35–42.

[19] Tosti A, Piraccini BM, Alagna G. Temporary hair loss simulating alopecia areata after endovascular

surgery of cerebral arteriovenous malformations: a report of 3 cases. Arch Dermatol 1999;135: 1555–6.

[20] Tosti A, Piraccini BM, Vincenzi C, et al. Permanent alopecia after busulfan chemotherapy. Br J Dermatol 2005;152:1056–8.

[21] Wolf R, Matz H, Zalish M, et al. Prostaglandin analogs for hair growth: great expectations. Dermatol Online J 2003;9:7.

[22] Peluso AM, Misciali C, Vincenzi C, et al. Diffuse hypertrichosis during treatment with 5% topical minoxidil. Br J Dermatol 1997;136:118–20.

[23] Grevelman EG, Breed WP. Prevention of chemotherapy-induced hair loss by scalp cooling. Ann Oncol 2005;16:352–8.

[24] Duvic M, Lemak NA, Valero V, et al. A randomized trial of minoxidil in chemotherapy-induced alopecia. J Am Acad Dermatol 1996;35:74–8.

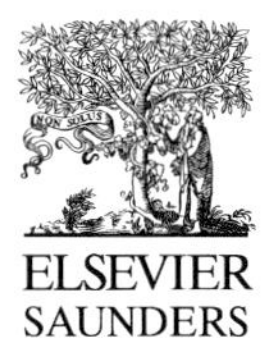

ELSEVIER
SAUNDERS

Dermatol Clin 25 (2007) 233–244

DERMATOLOGIC
CLINICS

Drug-Associated Lymphoma and Pseudolymphoma: Recognition and Management

Joerg Albrecht, MD[a], Lauren Ann Fine, MD[a], Warren Piette, MD[a,b,*]

[a]Department of Medicine, Division of Dermatology, John Stroger Jr. Hospital of Cook County, Administration Bldg., 1900 W Polk Street, Chicago, IL 60612, USA
[b]Department of Dermatology, Rush Medical Center, 1653 W Congress Parkway, Chicago, IL 60612, USA

Over the last 30 years, the classification of pseudolymphomas and lymphomas has undergone significant change, especially following the application of sophisticated immunostaining and gene rearrangement analysis. The term cutaneous pseudolymphomas (CPL) is a nonspecific term for a heterogeneous group of benign reactive T- or B-cell lymphoproliferative processes that simulate cutaneous lymphomas clinically or histologically. While pseudolymphomas are relatively rare, their clinical and histological heterogeneity has led to multiple systems of categorization based on immunological factors, causative agents, presentation, and clinical course. Some terms for cutaneous pseudolymphoma include:

Lymphadenosis benigna cutis (Bäfverstedt)
Cutaneous lymphoid hyperplasia (nodular or bandlike and perivascular pattern)
Lymphocytoma cutis
Sarcomatosis Spiegler-Fendt
Bäfverstedt syndrome
Kaposi-Spiegler sarcomatosis
Miliary lymphocytoma
Sarcomatosis cutis

This article focuses on lymphomas and pseudolymphomas associated with drug exposure.

Before the advent of immunophenotyping and immunogenetic analysis, classification was primarily based on morphological criteria and clinical findings (eg, the benign clinical course of pseudolymphomas). Detailed immunohistochemical and genetic analysis has led to the understanding that cutaneous lymphomas and pseudolymphomas are polar extremes of a spectrum, rather than strictly separate diseases. Supporting this understanding are clinical observations that demonstrate the transformation of pseudolymphomas into lymphomas. This transformation cannot accurately be predicted by the presence of a monoclonal infiltrate.

In most cases, the cause of pseudolymphomas remains unknown. Some are associated with photosensitivity, but various triggers beyond medications have been implicated. Suspected potential triggers include foreign agents, such as tattoo dye, bites, scabies, arthropod venom, contactants (eg, gold earrings), and hyposensitivity injections. Infectious agents have also been implicated, including HIV, varicella zoster virus, and *Borrelia burgdorferi*. In some areas, particularly in Europe, *B burgdorferi* is such a dominant cause of B-cell pseudolymphomas that antibiotic treatment is recommended as routine therapy if other obvious causes are not identified [1].

Pseudolymphomas affecting the skin can be divided clinically into two categories: (1) acute systemic syndromes and (2) subacute or chronic cases that primarily or exclusively involve the skin. The pseudolymphomas more familiar to non-dermatologists are systemic syndromes presenting with fever, eosinophilia, circulating atypical lymphocytes, and, often, lymphadenopathy and multiorgan involvement. Cutaneous involvement is often prominent and is typically among the

---

* Corresponding author. Department of Medicine, Division of Dermatology, John Stroger Jr. Hospital of Cook County, Administration Bldg., Rm. 519, 1900 W. Polk St., Chicago, IL 60612.

E-mail address: wpiette@cchil.org (W. Piette).

0733-8635/07/$ - see front matter © 2007 Elsevier Inc. All rights reserved.
doi:10.1016/j.det.2007.01.008

presenting signs, but is usually nonspecific. However, histologic changes mimicking lymphoma are usually found only in the lymph nodes and only rarely in the skin in these syndromes. Progression of some patients to systemic lymphoma has been reported [2–4]. Many terms have been used for this syndrome type. Some are listed in Table 1 [5–7]. Some authors include Stevens-Johnson syndrome or toxic epidermal necrolysis, provided the systemic symptoms are present, but this use is not generally accepted [8].

The second category of skin-related pseudolymphomas includes those in which the cutaneous histologic findings and even the clinical presentation mimic either B- or T-cell lymphomas. Findings are typically limited to the skin. Instances of progression from this form of pseudolymphoma to lymphoma have also been reported, but many of these precede the advent of current multifaceted tissue diagnostic techniques. Rather than progression to lymphoma, at least some of these cases may be examples of the indolent course of primary cutaneous lymphomas, especially B-cell lymphoma, which remain diagnostic challenges, particularly early in the course of disease.

Historical aspects and evolution of terminology

The evolution of thinking regarding cutaneous pseudolymphomas started in 1891, when patients with these findings were first reported as sarcomatosis cutis by Kaposi. In 1894, Spiegler described cutaneous lymphoid hyperplasia in patients who presented with the clinical features of a sarcoma but experienced a benign clinical course. In 1923, Biberstein coined the term lymphocytoma cutis, followed in 1943 by Bäfverstedt's emphasis on the benign character of the lesions by proposing the term lymphadenosis benigna cutis. The first use of the term pseudolymphoma in Pubmed can be found in an article from 1963 and refers to a gastric pseudolymphoma [9]. In 1967 Lever introduced the term "pseudolymphoma of Spiegler and Fendt" [10]. The existence of cutaneous T-cell pseudolymphomas was not widely accepted until the 1980s.

Drug-induced pseudolymphomas were first described based on experience with phenytoin (diphenylhydantion). Hypersensitivity reactions to phenytoin can be traced back to the year it was synthesized, 1908, when the drug was used to treat Sydenham chorea [11]. In 1938, the drug was first used to control seizures, and 2 years later the first hydantoin-induced lymphadenopathy was reported. In 1959, Saltzstein and Ackerman [12] described anticonvulsant-induced lymphadenopathy that mimicked malignant lymphoma. In 1970, Anthony [13] published evidence of an increased incidence of lymphoma in phenytoin users. The syndrome was renamed anticonvulsant hypersensitivity syndrome in 1988 as it became clear that anticonvulsants other than phenytoin could cause the same symptoms [11]. Drugs that often cause this syndrome, apart from anticonvulsants, are sulfonamides and allopurinol [14].

Classification/histology

Pseudolymphomas can be categorized according to histology, molecular markers, etiology, and clinical characteristics. One suggestion for classification can be found in Box 1.

Histological classification

In the 1980s, Burg and Braun-Falco based their classification of cutaneous pseudolymphomas on

Table 1
Terms used to describe hypersensitivity syndrome

Name	Pubmed hits (search term)
Anticonvulsant hypersensitivity syndrome [76]	74 ("anticonvulsant hypersensitivity syndrome")
Pseudolymphoma syndrome [43]	14 ("pseudolymphoma syndrome")
Drug-induced delayed multiorgan hypersensitivity syndrome (DIDMOHS) [5]	2 (DIDMOHS)
Drug rash with eosinophilia and systemic symptoms (DRESS) [2]	43 (DRESS + eosinophilia)
Drug hypersensitivity syndrome (DHS) [4,8]	64 ("drug hypersensitivity syndrome")
Idiosyncratic drug hypersensitivity syndrome [6]	1 ("idiosyncratic drug hypersensitivity syndrome")
Kawasaki-like syndrome [7]	5 ("Kawasaki-like" and drug cause given)
Cutaneous pseudolymphoma	50 ("cutaneous pseudolymphoma")

Box 1. Classification of pseudolymphoma according to histology and etiology

Bandlike cutaneous T-cell pseudolymphoma (major pattern)
Idiopathic
Lymphomatoid drug eruption
Nodular scabies (minority of scabies cases)
Actinic reticuloid
Lymphomatoid papulosis (type B, rare)
Clonal cutaneous T-cell pseudolymphoma
Lymphomatoid contact dermatitis

Nodular cutaneous T-cell pseudolymphoma (minor pattern)
Anticonvulsant-induced pseudolymphoma syndrome
Persistent nodular arthropod bites
Nodular scabies (majority of scabies cases)
Acral pseudolymphoma angiokeratoma
Lymphomatoid papulosis (types A and C)

Cutaneous B-cell pseudolymphomas (nodular pattern)
Idiopathic lymphocytoma cutis
Borrelial lymphocytoma cutis
Tattoo-induced lymphocytoma cutis
Post-herpes zoster scar lymphocytoma cutis
Lymphocytoma cutis by silver injection/acupuncture
Persistent nodular arthropod-bite reactions
Lymphomatoid drug eruptions
Acral pseudolymphoma angiokeratoma
Clonal cutaneous B-cell pseudolymphoma

Modified from Ploysangam T, Breneman DL, Mutasim DF. Cutaneous pseudolymphomas. J Am Acad Dermatol 1998;38(6 Pt 1):877–95.

---

the immunohistochemical differentiation between cutaneous T-cell pseudolymphomas (CTPL) and cutaneous B-cell pseudolymphomas (CBPL) and their histologic patterns. The pattern is either bandlike and superficial (like mycosis fungoides) or nodular in CTPL, but almost exclusively nodular in CBPL. Differences in histology and etiology between these groups are highlighted in Box 1. Accurate histologic differentiation of pseudolymphomas requires a deep biopsy that includes subcutaneous fat.

In the anticonvulsant-induced pseudolymphoma syndrome, lymph-node changes with focal necrosis, eosinophilic and histiocytic cell infiltrates, and destruction of node architecture have been described. However, Reed-Sternberg cells are not found [10].

Jessner's lymphocytic infiltrate has occasionally been categorized as a pseudolymphoma, but its description does not include atypical lymphocytes or lymphoid follicles, and its existence as a distinct entity is controversial [10,15].

Cutaneous T-cell pseudolymphomas

Mycosis fungoides–like pseudolymphomas are the most frequent drug-induced pseudolymphomas [16]. A superficial bandlike infiltrate of mostly small T cells in the papillary dermis may blur the epidermal junction. Epidermotropism of the lymphocytes is variable; sometimes Pautrier microabcesses can be found. The extent of acanthosis varies; spongiosis tends to be minimal. Polymorphous infiltrates may be found in deep perivascular or periadnexal locations.

Nodular drug-induced CTPLs that mimic non-Hodgkin's lymphomas or CBPL occur rarely, and may coexist in patients with mycosis fungoides–like lesions. The infiltrate demonstrates minimal or no atypia with small lymphocytes and variable histiocytes, plasma cells, or eosinophils.

Cutaneous B-cell pseudolymphomas

Nodular drug-induced CBPL is uncommon to rare. It presents histologically with nodules containing mildly atypical lymphocytes interspersed with a variety of mononuclear cells. An infiltrate containing well-formed germinal centers limited to papillary and upper reticular dermis (top heavy) favors pseudolymphoma. Rarely, the infiltrate extends into the subcutaneous fat and mimics a cutaneous B-cell lymphoma (bottom heavy). Drug-induced lymphomas may be localized or, rarely, generalized [17].

Differentiation of pseudolymphoma from lymphoma

Before the advent of immunophenotyping and immunoglobulin and T-cell receptor gene arrangement analysis, the diagnosis of pseudolymphomas was primarily based on histology and lack of systemic involvement within 5 years after diagnosis [10]. However, some pseudolymphomas, particularly those induced by anticonvulsants, demonstrate significant systemic symptoms from the onset, in spite of their benign course.

The confusion regarding the nosology of pseudolymphomas and its relationship with other lymphoproliferative disorders is based partly on their occasionally erratic clinical course with transformation into T-cell lymphomas. This apparent transformation may be due to either initial misdiagnosis or genuine transformation to or replacement by a lymphoma. Some of these reports of transformations predate current diagnostic standards [18].

The differentiation between drug-induced cutaneous lymphomas or pseudolymphomas relies primarily on clinical evaluation, light microscopy, clonality analysis, and immunohistochemistry.

T-cell pseudolymphomas

Clinical presentations

In the differentiation of pseudolymphoma from cutaneous lymphomas, the clinical history is of primary importance. Characteristics of mycosis fungoides are the presence of lesions in sun-protected areas, such as the buttocks; multiple and varied morphology of lesions; and a prolonged clinical history without regression. Pseudolymphoma, particularly if its onset is delayed after the initiation of drug therapy, more frequently presents with singular lesions and, if multiple, are often of similar morphology and without a sun-protected site localization. However, monolesional mycosis fungoides has been observed [19]. In some cases of lichen sclerosus the diagnosis may be challenging without clinicopathologic correlation because the disease may present with mycosis fungoides–like pseudolymphomatous histological features [20].

Atypical pigmentary purpura, resembling lichen aureus or, more often, Schamberg's purpura, may be a presentation of mycosis fungoides but may also be a reversible drug-induced syndrome [21]. Interestingly, among the patients in this study who had polymerase chain reaction analysis for clonality, two drug-related and two idiopathic pigmentary purpura cases without mycosis fungoides demonstrated clonality, while the two cases of mycosis fungoides–related pigmentary purpura did not.

Light microscopy

Even light microscopy may show some differences between mycosis fungoides and its drug-induced mimics. The lymphocytic infiltrate is, in general, polymorphic, even if the mycosis fungoides pattern is present. Pseudolymphomas demonstrate frequent dermal infiltration while mycosis fungoides is more epidermotropic [22]. A more detailed comparison of the histologic features of mycosis fungoides–like pseudolymphoma and mycosis fungoides is provided in Table 2.

Clonality

As a general rule, lymphomas reveal a monoclonal population of lymphocytes while the pseudolymphomas show polyclonal infiltrates. The detection of clonality is usually done by polymerase chain reaction, which is able to identify a clonal population comprising as little as 1% of the lymphocytic infiltrate [23]. Clonality has been advocated as a diagnostic test for lymphoma despite a benign histologic appearance [24]. However, this technique can lead the clinician astray because >50% of patch-test lesions in one study as well as other benign dermatoses (eg, lichen planus, lichen sclerosus, or pityriasis lichenoides et varioliformis acuta) have demonstrated monoclonal infiltrates [20,23,25].

Immunohistochemistry

Immunohistochemistry of T-cell receptors has been advocated to differentiate mycosis fungoides

Table 2
Differential diagnostic signs to distinguish pseudolymphoma and mycosis fungoides

Histologic findings	Pseudolymphoma	Mycosis fungoides
Epidermis		
Spongiosis	Moderate to severe	Absent or minimal
Necrotic keratinocytes	Common	Rare
Epithelial infiltration	Frequent but mild	Rare
Atypical epidermal lymphocytes	Polymorphic	Monomorphic
Dermis		
Papillary dermal edema	Very common	Rare
Extravasation of erythocytes	Very common	Rare
Mixed cell infiltrate	Common	Uncommon
Mitosis	Many	A few
Size of lymphocytes	Dermal > epidermal	Epidermal > dermal
Papillary dermal fibrosis	Rare	Rule

from benign conditions. However, the use of heterodimers of the constant regions have produced disappointing results since immunophenotype characteristic of early mycosis fungoides and benign skin lesions reflect the vast majority of mature peripheral T cells: CD3+, TCR-beta+, and TCR-delta−, in both conditions [26].

Monoclonality of the variable region has not been universally successful, nor has T-cell receptor gene rearrangement. Both investigations demonstrated polyclonality in mycosis fungoides as well as monoclonality in benign conditions. Previous series have detected monoclonality in a variety of benign skin conditions with a frequency of up to 6% [27]. In a smaller series, Choi and colleagues [28] demonstrated a case of monoclonal infiltrate in a pseudolymphoma secondary to valproate. The difficulty of finding a monoclonal population of T cells in early mycosis fungoides may be due to the limited number of neoplastic lymphocytes in the early phases of the disease. Microdissection may be helpful to increase the sensitivity of the diagnosis of mycosis fungoides [23].

Another proposed marker of mycosis fungoides is a CD4/8 ratio of >4:1. However, in a series of drug-induced pseudolymphoma, Magro and colleagues [29] found a similar ratio in most cases, rendering this investigation useless to differentiate these two diseases.

As an expression of malignant transformation, neoplastic lymphocytes in mycosis fungoides are characterized by frequent deletions of the pan–T-cell markers CD7 and CD62K. Expression of <50% CD7 and CD62K has been suggested to indicate mycosis fungoides [29]. However, in 16 of 19 drug-induced pseudolymphomas, Magro and colleagues [29] demonstrated CD7 expression of <50% and significant reduction of CD62K in 2 cases. This reduction in receptor expression is also typical for memory T cells [29].

In the skin, anaplastic large cell lymphoma (ALCL) and lymphomatoid papulosis are characterized by the expression of CD30 antigen while mycosis fungoides is usually not. However large CD30+ T cells have been observed in several reactive conditions, including drug eruptions. Unlike in ALCL, CD30+ cells in reactive lesions are present only in small numbers, are scattered throughout, and are not arranged in clusters or sheets [23]. In general, the admixture of B and T cells with CD30+ cells seems to suggest a benign process.

B-cell pseudolymphomas

Clinical information

In general, B-cell pseudolymphomas present as singular lesions, though drug-induced pseudolymphomas are often multiple [23]. They also tend to occur at a younger age and a provoking agent may be suggested by careful history [22]. B-cell lymphomas present as clusters of irregularly shaped papules and nodules surrounded by erythematous patches and plaques, which typically affect the head, neck, and back. As associated symptoms of pseudolymphomas, Bence-Jones proteinuria and hypergammaglobulinemia may be observed, and may be reversible on discontinuation of the drug [30].

Light microscopy

Characteristically, monomorphic follicles indicate CBCL, but marginal zone lymphoma may have mixed cell infiltrates with eosinophils and small granulomas, which may be impossible to differentiate from pseudolymphomas on histopathology alone.

Clonality

Monoclonal arrangement of immunoglobulin heavy- and light-chain genes seems to differentiate well between CBCL and drug-induced CBPL [23].

Immunohistochemistry

There are various immunohistochemical criteria that have been tested to differentiate CBCL and CBPLs. Analysis of the immunoglobulin light-chain pattern has been used but restrictions of immunoglobulin seen in CBCL are not particularly helpful. Immunoglobulin negative B-cell proliferations seem to be particularly high in CBPL, making differentiation from CBCL difficult [23]. CD10+ and BCL6 can be found outside the follicles in CBCL, while in CBPL these cells are confined to the germinal centers [23]. Also, compared to follicle center cell lymphomas, reactive CBPL show higher activity of Ki-67/MIB-1 [23]. Detection of aberrant phenotypes of B-cell lymphomas (CD20+, CD5+, CD43+) are considered a sign of malignancy [23].

Clinical course, signs, and symptoms

Clinical course

Characteristically, anticonvulsant-induced pseudolymphoma-hypersensitivity syndromes develop soon after the drug has been started, usually within 2 to 8 weeks [31]. However, cases have developed as early as 5 days [10] and as late as 7 years [27]. Skin lesions and systemic symptoms resolve after discontinuing offending agents, usually within 3 to 4 weeks [10,32]. In one series, for pseudolymphomas without systemic symptoms, the resolution of the accompanying lymphadenopathy took 3 to 6 months [4]. This general picture contrasts with true lymphoma, which usually develops over several years and characteristically does not improve after discontinuation of the drug [18,31]. Reports have described pseudo-pseudolymphomas that regressed after discontinuation of phenytoin, with occurrence of a fatal lymphoma months later [33]. Even localized pseudolymphoma may return after a number of years in a different location [4]. These clinical settings suggest that long-term follow-up of patients is needed to assure the absence of lymphoproliferative malignancy [34,35].

Acute drug-induced hypersensitivity syndrome may have a mortality of 10%. This is largely independent of skin involvement and mostly due to liver or cardiac failure [14].

Hypersensitivity syndrome

The classic systemic hypersensitivity syndrome, as opposed to localized pseudolymphomas, was described first with anticonvulsants. Most patients with anticonvulsant-induced pseudolymphoma have systemic disease. This systemic disease develops with high-spiking fever, hepatomegaly, and localized or systemic lymphadenopathy, often with grape-sized nodes [36]. Severely abnormal liver function is a poor prognostic indicator and other organs, such as the gastrointestinal tract, the heart, or the lungs, can be involved. Usually the fever is the first symptom with skin findings developing later [8]. A variety of hematological abnormalities have been described in relationship with the syndrome. Most commonly, eosinophilia is observed but leucocytosis with increased T-cell count and atypical lymphocytes, neutrophilia, monocytosis, and aplastic anemia are also found. Circulating Sézary cells may make the clinical pathological and immunological differentiation from Sézary syndrome difficult [34].

A recent review of the literature and a large French database summarizing the characteristics of 446 cases demonstrated a variety of symptoms with skin findings predominating and frequent fever, blood abnormalities, and hepatic involvement [3]. The skin manifestations can appear as a single lesion, but a minority of patients have widespread erythematous papules, plaques, or nodules [14], which can progress to exfoliative dermatitis. Pustular variations, which may generalize [37], are frequent, as is edema, particularly of the face. The patients may develop conjunctivitis, pharyngitis, and a strawberry tongue [36].

Cutaneous pseudolymphoma with minimal systemic symptoms

The cutaneous pseudolymphomas with minimal to no systemic involvement often begin insidiously as cutaneous erythematous nodule and plaque formation several months after initiation of the offending drug. These cutaneous lesions demonstrate histologic pseudolymphoma and resolve usually after discontinuation of the drug. Some patients may have an increased likelihood of lymphomatous transformation later in life. These patients do not have fever, but may have lymphadenopathy and, possibly, hepatomegaly. Blood abnormalities, such as atypical lymphocytes or Sézary cells, can also be observed [4].

Pathophysiology

The pathophysiology of pseudolymphomas is not understood. It certainly is a multifactorial process dependent not just on drug exposure but also on other unknown cofactors [8]. Initially, pseudolymphomas were thought to be a pure hypersensitivity reaction, but the prevalent model is an immune dysregulation with a combination of immunosuppression, reduced immunosurveillance, and an abnormal proliferation of T lymphocytes and hypergammaglobuninaemia.

Several of the offending drugs, such as anticonvulsants, antidepressants, phenothiazines, angiotensin-converting enzyme inhibitors, and antihistamines, perturb lymphoid function in vitro and may promote blast transformation and impair T-cell suppressor function to induce an exaggerated lymphocyte response to exogenous antigenic triggers [29]. Lymphoma genesis is a stepwise process that begins with chronic immune stimulation as a trigger coupled with immune dysregulation [29]. This may well be caused by the offending drugs as a drug-induced dysregulated immune reaction to the drug itself or to some other drug or nonpharmacological antigen [38]. This theory is supported by some in vivo evidence of disturbance of the immune system by the offending drugs. Examples of such evidence include precipitation of lupus erythematosus by antihistamines and β-antagonists and -blockers or hyporeactivity in delayed-type hypersensitivity skin tests secondary to calcium channel blockers. Also the combination of immunomodulating drugs has a synergistic effect on suppression of T-lymphocyte function even if the mode of each agent is different [38]. This interaction among drugs is magnified if there is also drug metabolism interference [38], explaining the higher risk of pseudolymphoma in slow acetylators [39].

Positive patch tests and lymphocyte stimulation tests in patients with severe carbamazepine hypersensitivity indicate specific T-cell reactivity in these patients [40]. Positive patch tests have also been found in hypersensitivity syndromes secondary to other drugs, indicating that this phenomenon is not limited to carbamazepine [41]. Pseudolymphomas of the lymphomatoid contact dermatitis type are rare but well described and associated with positive patch tests [42]. Also, in a minority of cases of drug-induced pseudolymphoma, intraepidermal CD8-positive lymphocytes were found, while the dermal lymphocyte population was primarily CD4, suggesting a pattern typical of type IV immune reaction with combined delayed-type hypersensitivity and cellular cytotoxic features [29]. Findings of deleted CD7 and CD62K activated memory T cells have led to the term "drug-induced reversible lymphoid dyscrasia" to describe an unrepressed expansion of lymphocytes in response to an antigenic trigger [29].

CD30- and CD4-expressing lymphocytes accentuated around blood vessels and acrosyringia—the latter a site of preferential antigen processing—are other clues to antigenic stimulation as a trigger for an atypical lymphocytic infiltrate.

The increased incidence of Hodgkin's and non-Hodgkin's lymphomas described after phenyotin therapy, and sometimes following pseudolymphomas [13], could be explained by persistent antigenic stimulation and rise of autonomous lymphocyte clones in a state of immunogenic imbalance [43].

Another theory is based on possible cell damage with hapten generation secondary to drug metabolites, which in turn generates an immune response. It is thought that offending drugs metabolize to highly reactive arene oxide or epioxide metabolites or other metabolites formed by cytochrome P450 enzymes or by myeloperoxidase. These may bind to tissue macromolecules and cause cell damage. Arene metabolites, which are metabolites of the aromatic rings of many anticonvulsants, have in vitro been elegantly shown to elicit lymphocytic responses [44]. These similar metabolic products may explain the clearly observed cross-reactivity between different aromatic anticonvulsants [45,46]. The relevance of metabolic processes is supported by the observation that first-degree relatives are at increased risk of developing similar hypersensitivity syndromes [46], and again by the higher risk for slow acetylators [2,39]. A reduction of the starting dose of lamotrigene has been shown to virtually eliminate serious cutaneous drug reactions. One explanation suggested was that the drug level was below a certain threshold necessary to elicit this kind of serious drug reaction [47]. However, cross-reactivity has also been observed between two angiotensin receptor antagonists that were structurally unrelated [16].

As mentioned above, some of the theories for the pathophysiology of pseudolymphoma implicate cofactors that may help to induce the disease. HIV patients have been shown to have higher incidence of serious drug reactions [8]. Recent publications suggest that herpes simplex virus 6 (HHV 6) reactivation may be associated with drug rash with eosinophilia and systemic symptoms [48–50]. However, given that the seroprevalence of HHV 6 nears 100% and that not all patients had positive HHV 6 IgM titers, the proof of a causative role is lacking.

Drugs implicated in pseudolymphoma

The number of drugs implicated in pseudolymphomas or hypersensitivity syndrome is constantly rising and thus Box 2 can only give some guidance of the range of drugs implicated. The identification of these drugs is further complicated by the nomenclature used to describe the clinical symptoms of pseudolymphomas, which may actually be based on the predominantly affected organ or the most life-threatening organ involvement [2]. The drugs in Box 2 [51–75] most commonly associated with pseudolymphoma or hypersensitivity syndromes are the aromatic anticonvulsants (eg, phenytoin, phenobarbital (phenobarbitone), and carbamazepine), lamotrigine [76], the sulfonamides, and allopurinol [14].

Epidemiology

No data is available on the overall incidence and prevalence of drug-induced pseudolymphoma. Adverse cutaneous reactions to medication can be found in approximately 2% to 3% of hospitalized patients [77]. The general incidence of drug-induced hypersensitivity syndrome can be estimated to be between 1 in 1000 to 1 in 10,000 patients exposed to anticonvulsants [78], or even up to 1 in 100 if any idiosyncratic hypersensitivity is counted [8]. The likelihood of 1 in 5000 patients, with a higher incidence in black patients, has been suggested based on the available evidence for anticonvulsants [14]. In a cohort of 8,888 new phenytoin users, there were 8 serious cutaneous reactions, including 2 probable and 2 possible cases of drug hypersensitivity syndrome, yielding a risk of 2.3 to 4.5 per 10,000. There were 6 serious cutaneous reactions in 9,738 new carbamazepine users, including 1 probable case and 4 possible cases, yielding a risk of 1 to 4.1 per 10,000 for this syndrome. No confirmed serious cutaneous diagnoses were observed in 1,504

new valproate users [79]. In general, black patients seem to be at a higher risk than white patients [10]. Slow acetylation is also thought to be a risk factor [39]. For CBPL, drug-induced or others, the male/female ratio is about 2:1. It is primarily a disease of the white population, occurring at a ratio of 9:1 compared with the black population. CBPL is a disease of early adulthood. The median age of patients with CBPL is about 34 years and >60% of the patients are younger than 40 years at the time of the initial biopsy [10]. Occurrence of phenytoin hypersensitivity syndrome in three siblings raises the possibility of genetic predisposition [80].

Evaluation and treatment of patients with pseudolymphoma

If an association with drug exposure is suspected, the most important therapeutic step is the discontinuation of the offending drug. This is true for all drug-induced diseases. Discontinuation alone is most often sufficient to lead to remission and confirms the etiology. Exposure to the same drug leads to severe reappearance of all symptoms [2].

Systemic corticosteroids (>0.5 mg/kg of body weight) are often used in the acute phase of acute hypersensitivity syndrome and have been described as having dramatic success if organs other than the skin are involved [2,14]. Rapid tapering of the corticosteroid dose can lead to reactivation of the disease [39], with improvement when the drug dose is increased [81]. This indicates that in at least some cases the use of corticosteroids is vital for accelerated resolution of the disease. Due to the possible reactivation of viruses, particularly herpes simplex 6 virus, it seems most prudent to restrict systemic corticosteroids to the most severe cases [39]. In cases where the lesions are secondary to contact dermatitis, the resolution can be hastened by topical corticosteroid use [10]. Most lesions of pseudolymphomas not complicated by systemic symptoms are not symptomatic and thus aggressive treatment is not mandated. Systemic and topical corticosteroids have been tried with mixed success.

Treatment of fever and pruritus is symptomatic. However, due to their hepatotoxicity, antipyretics, such as acetaminophen, should be used cautiously. Because development of lymphomas has been observed even in cases that demonstrated full clinical remission, long-term follow-up seems prudent.

Box 2. Drugs implicated in pseudolymphoma or hypersensitivity syndrome

Anticonvulsants [10,31,36,43,51,52]
  Phenytoin
  Carbamazepine
  Butabarbital
  Ethosuximide
  Lamotrigin
  Mephenytoin
  Methsuximide
  Phenobarbital
  Phensuximide
  Primidone
  Trimethadione

Antiarrhythmics [10,31]
  Mexiletine
  Procainamide

Antibiotics [10,14,41,53,54]
  Minocycline [but histology nonspecific dermal
    infiltrate]
  Cefixime
  Flucloxacillin
  Nitrofurantoin
  Penicillin
  Sulfonamides

Anticoagulants [55]
  Fluindione

Antidepressants [10,31,56]
  Amitriptyline
  Desipramine
  Doxepin
  Fluoxetine
  Lithium
  Maprotiline
  Thioridazine

Antihistamines [10,31]
  Cimetidine
  Diphenhydramine
  Ranitidine

Antihypertensives
  Alpha agonists [57]
    Clonidine patch

  Angiotensin-converting enzyme inhibitors
    [38,58,59]
    Benazepril
    Captopril
    Enalapril
    Lisinopril

  Angiotensin receptor blockers [16,60]
    Losartan
    Valsartan

β-Blockers [10,27,29,61]
  Atenolol
  Labetalol

Calcium channel blockers [10]
  Diltiazem
  Verapamil

Diuretics [10]
  Hydrochlorothiazide

Antipsychotics (phenothiazines) [10,31,62,78]
  Chlorpromazine
  Promethazine
  Levopromazine
  Thioridazine

Antirheumatics [10,31,38,63–67]
  Allopurinol
  D-penicillamine
  Gold
  Sulfasalazine
  Nonsteroidal anti-inflammatory drugs

Antiretrovirals [8,68]
  Abacavir
  Nevirapine

Antithyroid drug [69]
  Methimazole

Chemotherapeutics [15,30,70,71]
  Cyclosporine
  Glatiramer acetate
  Imatinib mesylate (Gleevec)
  Methotrexate

Cholesterol-lowering drugs/3-hydroxy-3-
  methylglutaryl coenzyme A reductase
  inhibitors [10,38]
  Lovastatin

Fillers [72]
  Silicone injection

Sedatives [10]
  Clonazepam
  Lorazepam

Sex steroids [10,38]
  Estrogen
  Progesterone

Topical agents [10,73]
  Etheric plant oil
  Hydroquinone cream
  Menthol

Vaccines [74,75]
  Hepatitis A or B vaccine injection sites

Cryosurgery, laser ablation, surgical excision, and radiotherapy have been tried. Radiotherapy has been used particularly in treating facial lesions that cannot be satisfactorily removed surgically. Invasive surgical approaches should only be used if the lesion does not resolve after discontinuation of the potentially offending drug.

Summary

The occurrence of pseudolymphomas in patients receiving anticonvulsants and other drugs is uncommon. However, clinicians must be prepared to recognize such pseudolymphomas. Management consists mainly in discontinuation of the offending agent and symptomatic treatment in the acutely ill. Careful drug history is necessary in all patients who develop atypical cutaneous infiltrates, and most patients show improvement within several weeks after drug discontinuation. Failure of lesions to resolve months after drug modulation should raise suspicion for a malignant process and trigger appropriate investigations.

References

[1] Kaudewitz P. Pseudolymphomas of the skin (Pseudolymphome der Haut). In: Braun-Falko O, Plewig G, Wolff HH, editors. Dermatology and venerology (Dermatologie und Venerologie). Berlin: Springer; 1996. p. 1390–6.

[2] Bocquet H, Bagot M, Roujeau JC. Drug-induced pseudolymphoma and drug hypersensitivity syndrome (Drug Rash with Eosinophilia and Systemic Symptoms: DRESS). Semin Cutan Med Surg 1996; 15(4):250–7.

[3] Peyrière H, Dereure O, Breton H, et al. Variability in the clinical pattern of cutaneous side-effects of drugs with systemic symptoms: does a DRESS syndrome really exist? Br J Dermatol 2006;155(2):422–8.

[4] Callot V, Roujeau JC, Bagot M, et al. Drug-induced pseudolymphoma and hypersensitivity syndrome. Two different clinical entities. Arch Dermatol 1996; 132(11):1315–21.

[5] Sontheimer RD, Houpt KR. DIDMOHS: a proposed consensus nomenclature for the drug-induced delayed multiorgan hypersensitivity syndrome. Arch Dermatol 1998;134(7):874–6.

[6] Bonnetblanc JM. Drug hypersensitivity syndrome. Dermatology 1993;187(2):84–5.

[7] Hicks RA, Murphy JV, Jackson MA. Kawasaki-like syndrome caused by carbamazepine. Pediatr Infect Dis J 1988;7(7):525–6.

[8] Sullivan JR, Shear NH. The drug hypersensitivity syndrome: what is the pathogenesis? Arch Dermatol 2001;137(3):357–64.

[9] Jacobs DS. Primary gastic malignant lymphoma and pseudolymphoma. Am J Clin Pathol 1963;40: 379–94.

[10] Ploysangam T, Breneman DL, Mutasim DF. Cutaneous pseudolymphomas. J Am Acad Dermatol 1998;38(6 Pt 1):877–95.

[11] Goel A, Walia RL. Pseudolymphoma revisited. Indian J Dermatol Venereol Leprol 2004;70:48–51.

[12] Salzstein SL, Ackerman LV. Lymphadenopathy induced by anticonvulsant drugs and mimicking clinically and pathologically malignant lymphoma. Cancer 1959;12:164–82.

[13] Anthony JJ. Malignant lymphoma associated with hydantoin drugs. Arch Neurol 1970;22(5):450–4.

[14] Roujeau JC, Stern RS. Severe adverse cutaneous reactions to drugs. N Engl J Med 1994;331(19): 1272–85.

[15] Nolden S, Casper C, Kuhn A, et al. Jessner-Kanof lymphocytic infiltration of the skin associated with glatiramer acetate. Mult Scler 2005;11(2):245–8.

[16] Mutasim DF. Lymphomatoid drug eruption mimicking digitate dermatosis: cross reactivity between two drugs that suppress angiotensin II function. Am J Dermatopathol 2003;25(4):331–4.

[17] Luelmo AJ, Mieras BC, Martin-Urda MT, et al. Generalized cutaneous B-cell pseudolymphoma induced by neuroleptics. Arch Dermatol 1992;128(1): 121–3.

[18] Hyman GA, Sommers SC. The development of Hodgkin's disease and lymphoma during anticonvulsant therapy. Blood 1966;28(3):416–27.

[19] Hodak E, Phenig E, Amichai B, et al. Unilesional mycosis fungoides: a study of seven cases. Dermatology 2000;201(4):300–6.

[20] Citarella L, Massone C, Kerl H, et al. Lichen sclerosus with histopathologic features simulating early mycosis fungoides. Am J Dermatopathol 2003; 25(6):463–5.

[21] Crowson AN, Magro CM, Zahorchak R. Atypical pigmentary purpura: a clinical, histopathologic, and genotypic study. Hum Pathol 1999;30(9): 1004–12.

[22] Rijlaarsdam JU, Willemze R. Cutaneous pseudolymphomas: classification and differential diagnosis. Semin Dermatol 1994;13(3):187–96.

[23] Cerroni L, Goteri G. Differential diagnosis between cutaneous lymphoma and pseudolymphoma. Anal Quant Cytol Histol 2003;25(4):191–8.

[24] Flaig MJ, Cerroni L, Schuhmann K, et al. Follicular mycosis fungoides. A histopathologic analysis of nine cases. J Cutan Pathol 2001;28(10):525–30.

[25] Holm N, Flaig MJ, Yazdi AS, et al. The value of molecular analysis by PCR in the diagnosis of cutaneous lymphocytic infiltrates. J Cutan Pathol 2002; 29(8):447–52.

[26] Michie SA, Abel EA, Hoppe RT, et al. Expression of T-cell receptor antigens in mycosis fungoides and inflammatory skin lesions. J Invest Dermatol 1989; 93(1):116–20.

[27] Wood GS, Tung RM, Haeffner AC, et al. Detection of clonal T-cell receptor gamma gene rearrangements in early mycosis fungoides/Sezary syndrome by polymerase chain reaction and denaturing gradient gel electrophoresis (PCR/DGGE). J Invest Dermatol 1994;103(1):34–41.

[28] Choi TS, Doh KS, Kim SH, et al. Clinicopathological and genotypic aspects of anticonvulsant-induced pseudolymphoma syndrome. Br J Dermatol 2003; 148(4):730–6.

[29] Magro CM, Crowson AN, Kovatich AJ, et al. Drug-induced reversible lymphoid dyscrasia: a clonal lymphomatoid dermatitis of memory and activated T cells. Hum Pathol 2003;34(2):119–29.

[30] Delaporte E, Catteau B, Cardon T, et al. [Cutaneous pseudolymphoma during treatment of rheumatoid polyarthritis with low-dose methotrexate]. Ann Dermatol Venereol 1995;122(8):521–5 [in French].

[31] Kardaun SH, Scheffer E, Vermeer BJ. Drug-induced pseudolymphomatous skin reactions. Br J Dermatol 1988;118(4):545–52.

[32] Wolf R, Kahane E, Sandbank M. Mycosis fungoides-like lesions associated with phenytoin therapy. Arch Dermatol 1985;121(9):1181–2.

[33] Gams RA, Neal JA, Conrad FG. Hydantoin-induced pseudo-pseudolymphoma. Ann Intern Med 1968;69(3):557–68.

[34] D'Incan M, Souteyrand P, Bignon YJ, et al. Hydantoin-induced cutaneous pseudolymphoma with clinical, pathologic, and immunologic aspects of Sezary syndrome. Arch Dermatol 1992;128(10): 1371–4.

[35] Kulow BF, Cualing H, Steele P, et al. Progression of cutaneous B-cell pseudolymphoma to cutaneous B-cell lymphoma. J Cutan Med Surg 2002;6(6): 519–28.

[36] Harris DW, Ostlere L, Buckley C, et al. Phenytoin-induced pseudolymphoma. A report of a case and review of the literature. Br J Dermatol 1992;127(4): 403–6.

[37] Kleier RS, Breneman DL, Boiko S. Generalized pustulation as a manifestation of the anticonvulsant hypersensitivity syndrome. Arch Dermatol 1991; 127(9):1361–4.

[38] Magro CM, Crowson AN. Drug-induced immune dysregulation as a cause of atypical cutaneous lymphoid infiltrates: a hypothesis. Hum Pathol 1996; 27(2):125–32.

[39] Ghislain PD, Roujeau JC. Treatment of severe drug reactions: Steven-Johnsons syndrome, toxic epidermal necrolysis and hypersensitivity syndrome. Dermatol Online J 2002;8(1):5.

[40] Houwerzijl J, De Gast GC, Nater JP, et al. Lymphocyte-stimulation tests and patch tests to carbamazepine hypersensitivity. Clin Exp Immunol 1977;29(2):272–7.

[41] Antunes A, Davril A, Trechot P, et al. [Minocycline hypersensitivity syndrome]. Ann Dermatol Venereol 1999;126(6–7):518–21 [in French].

[42] Braun RP, French LE, Feldmann R, et al. Cutaneous pseudolymphoma, lymphomatoid contact dermatitis type, as an unusual cause of symmetrical upper eyelid nodules. Br J Dermatol 2000;143(2): 411–4.

[43] De Vriese AS, Philippe J, Van Renterghem DM, et al. Carbamazepine hypersensitivity syndrome: report of 4 cases and review of the literature. Medicine (Baltimore) 1995;74(3):144–51.

[44] Spielberg SP, Gordon GB, Blake DA, et al. Predisposition to phenytoin hepatotoxicity assessed in vitro. N Engl J Med 1981;305(13):722–7.

[45] Shear NH, Spielberg SP. Anticonvulsant hypersensitivity syndrome. In vitro assessment of risk. J Clin Invest 1988;82(6):1826–32.

[46] Nathan DL, Belsito DV. Carbamazepine-induced pseudolymphoma with CD-30 positive cells. J Am Acad Dermatol 1998;38(5 Pt 2):806–9.

[47] Wong IC, Mawer GE, Sander JW. Factors influencing the incidence of lamotrigine-related skin rash. Ann Pharmacother 1999;33(10):1037–42.

[48] Descamps V, Valance A, Edlinger C, et al. Association of human herpesvirus 6 infection with drug reaction with eosinophilia and systemic symptoms. Arch Dermatol 2001;137(3):301–4.

[49] Ichiche M, Kiesch N, De Bels D. DRESS syndrome associated with HHV-6 reactivation. Eur J Intern Med 2003;14(8):498–500.

[50] Debarbieux S, Deroo-Berger MC, Grande S, et al. [Drug hypersensitivity syndrome associated with a primary HHV6 infection]. Ann Dermatol Venereol 2006;133(2):145–7 [in French].

[51] Beller TC, Boyce JA. Prolonged anticonvulsant hypersensitivity syndrome related to lamotrigine in a patient with human immunodeficiency virus. Allergy Asthma Proc 2002;23(6):415–9.

[52] Masruha MR, Marques CM, Vilanova LC, et al. Drug induced pseudolymphoma secondary to ethosuximide. J Neurol Neurosurg Psychiatr 2005; 76(11):1610.

[53] Melzer M, Keane FM, Eykyn SJ, et al. A pseudolymphomatous skin reaction secondary to flucloxacillin. J Infect 2000;40(2):198–9.

[54] Jabbar A, Siddique T. A case of pseudolymphoma leukaemia syndrome following cefixime. Br J Haematol 1998;101(1):209.

[55] Frouin E, Roth B, Grange A, et al. [Hypersensitivity to fluindione (Previscan). Positive skin patch tests]. Ann Dermatol Venereol 2005;132(12 Pt 1):1000–2 [in French].

[56] Milionis HJ, Skopelitou A, Elisaf MS. Hypersensitivity syndrome caused by amitriptyline administration. Postgrad Med J 2000;76(896):361–3.

[57] Shelley WB, Shelley ED. Pseudolymphoma at site of clonidine patch. Lancet 1997;350(9086):1223–4.

[58] Wilkin JK, Hammond JJ, Kirkendall WM. The captopril-induced eruption. A possible mechanism: cutaneous kinin potentiation. Arch Dermatol 1980; 116(8):902–5.

[59] Furness PN, Goodfield MJ, MacLennan KA, et al. Severe cutaneous reactions to captopril and enalapril; histological study and comparison with early mycosis fungoides. J Clin Pathol 1986;39(8):902–7.

[60] Viraben R, Lamant L, Brousset P. Losartan-associated atypical cutaneous lymphoid hyperplasia. Lancet 1997;350(9088):1366.

[61] Henderson CA, Shamy HK. Atenolol-induced pseudolymphoma. Clin Exp Dermatol 1990;15(2):119–20.

[62] Blazejak T, Holzle E. [Phenothiazine-induced pseudolymphoma]. Hautarzt 1990;41(3):161–3 [in German].

[63] Raymond JZ, Goldman HM. An unusual cutaneous reaction secondary to allopurinol. Cutis 1988;41(5):323–6.

[64] Kim KJ, Lee MW, Choi JH, et al. CD30-positive T-cell-rich pseudolymphoma induced by gold acupuncture. Br J Dermatol 2002;146(5):882–4.

[65] Kalimo K, Rasanen L, Aho H, et al. Persistent cutaneous pseudolymphoma after intradermal gold injection. J Cutan Pathol 1996;23(4):328–34.

[66] Michel F, Navellou JC, Ferraud D, et al. DRESS syndrome in a patient on sulfasalazine for rheumatoid arthritis. Joint Bone Spine 2005;72(1):82–5.

[67] Teo L, Tan E. Sulphasalazine-induced DRESS. Singapore Med J 2006;47(3):237–9.

[68] Bourezane Y, Salard D, Hoen B, et al. DRESS (drug rash with eosinophilia and systemic symptoms) syndrome associated with nevirapine therapy. Clin Infect Dis 1998;27(5):1321–2.

[69] Ozaki N, Miura Y, Sakakibara A, et al. A case of hypersensitivity syndrome induced by methimazole for Graves' disease. Thyroid 2005;15(12):1333–6.

[70] Moseley AC, Lindsley HB, Skikne BS, et al. Reversible methotrexate associated lymphoproliferative disease evolving into Hodgkin's disease. J Rheumatol 2000;27(3):810–3.

[71] Clark SH, Duvic M, Prieto VG. Mycosis fungoides-like reaction in a patient treated with Gleevec. J Cutan Pathol 2003;30(4):279–81.

[72] Lee MW, Choi JH, Sung KJ, et al. A case of cutaneous pseudolymphoma associated with silicone injection. Acta Derm Venereol 2004;84(4):312–3.

[73] Dar NR, Shaheen, Mustafvi SA, et al. Cutaneous pseudolymphoma due to topical application of 4% hydroquinone cream for melasma. J Coll Physicians Surg Pak 2005;15(8):496–7.

[74] Maubec E, Pinquier L, Viguier M, et al. Vaccination-induced cutaneous pseudolymphoma. J Am Acad Dermatol 2005;52(4):623–9.

[75] Stavrianeas NG, Katoulis AC, Kanelleas A, et al. Papulonodular lichenoid and pseudolymphomatous reaction at the injection site of hepatitis B virus vaccination. Dermatology 2002;205(2):166–8.

[76] Knowles SR, Shapiro LE, Shear NH. Anticonvulsant hypersensitivity syndrome: incidence, prevention and management. Drug Saf 1999;21(6):489–501.

[77] Bigby M, Jick S, Jick H, et al. Drug-induced cutaneous reactions. A report from the Boston Collaborative Drug Surveillance Program on 15,438 consecutive inpatients, 1975 to 1982. JAMA 1986;256(24):3358–63.

[78] Knowles SR, Shapiro LE, Shear NH. Reactive metabolites and adverse drug reactions: clinical considerations. Clin Rev Allergy Immunol 2003;24(3):229–38.

[79] Tennis P, Stern RS. Risk of serious cutaneous disorders after initiation of use of phenytoin, carbamazepine, or sodium valproate: a record linkage study. Neurology 1997;49(2):542–6.

[80] Gennis MA, Vemuri R, Burns EA, et al. Familial occurrence of hypersensitivity to phenytoin. Am J Med 1991;91(6):631–4.

[81] Rekhtman D, Eisenstein EM. Glucocorticoid treatment of severe pediatric drug hypersensitivity syndrome. Pediatr Asthma Allerdgy Immunol 2005;18(3):156–60.

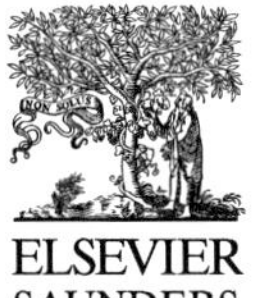

DERMATOLOGIC
CLINICS

Dermatol Clin 25 (2007) 245–253

Recognition and Management of Severe Cutaneous Drug Reactions

Sandra R. Knowles, BScPhm[a,c],
Neil H. Shear, MD, FRCPC, FACP[a,b,c],*

[a]*Faculty of Pharmacy, University of Toronto, 144 College Street, Toronto, ON M5S 3M2, Canada*
[b]*Dermatology, University of Toronto, Toronto, ON, Canada*
[c]*Sunnybrook Health Sciences Centre, Drug Safety Clinic,
2075 Bayview Avenue, Room M1 700, Toronto, ON M4N 3M5, Canada*

Cutaneous drug reactions are among the most common types of adverse drug reactions. This article focuses on the recognition and management of severe cutaneous drug eruptions, including the drug-hypersensitivity syndrome, serum sickness–like reaction, acute generalized exanthematous pustulosis (AGEP), Stevens-Johnson syndrome, and toxic epidermal necrolysis (Table 1). Cutaneous reactions are considered severe when they can result in serious skin damage or involve multiple organs. Some of these reactions can cause significant morbidity or death. Each may be confounded by diagnostic difficulties, confusion in ascertaining causality, and treatment challenges.

Recognition of severe cutaneous drug eruptions is difficult because they often occur in complicated clinical scenarios that may include exposure to multiple agents. New drugs, most often those started within the preceding 6 weeks, are potential causative agents (exceptions include drug-induced lupus, pemphigus, and pseudolymphoma), as are drugs that have been used intermittently, including over-the-counter preparations and herbal and naturopathic remedies.

Hypersensitivity syndrome

Hypersensitivity syndrome (also known as drug rash with eosinophilia and systemic symptoms or drug-induced hypersensitivity syndrome) is characterized by a triad of fever, skin eruption, and internal organ involvement. This syndrome has been well described for a number of drugs, including anticonvulsants, sulfonamide antibiotics, dapsone, minocycline, and allopurinol [1–3]. Although this reaction has been estimated to occur with a frequency of between 1 in 1000 and 1 in 10,000 anticonvulsant and sulfonamide antibiotic exposures, its true incidence is unknown because of variable presentation and inaccurate reporting [4]. Hypersensitivity syndrome occurs most frequently on first exposure to the drug, with initial symptoms starting 2 to 6 weeks after exposure to the drug. In patients with a history of hypersensitivity syndrome, reexposure to the offending agent may cause development of symptoms within 1 day. Hypersensitivity syndrome is not related to dose or serum concentration of the drug. The timing of onset and the clinical features vary among patients and vary among drugs. Often the syndrome is described with the preface of the name of the drug (eg, dapsone hypersensitivity syndrome).

A mild to high fever ranging from 38° to 40°C and malaise, which can be accompanied by pharyngitis and cervical lymphadenopathy, are the presenting symptoms in most patients. Atypical lymphocytosis with a subsequent prominent eosinophilia may occur during the initial phases of

* Corresponding author. Sunnybrook Health Sciences Centre, 2075 Bayview Avenue, Room M1 700, Toronto, ON M4N 3M5, Canada.

E-mail address: neil.shear@sunnybrook.ca (N.H. Shear).

0733-8635/07/$ - see front matter
doi:10.1016/j.det.2007.01.011

Table 1
Clinical features of drug-hypersensitivity syndrome, serum sickness–like reaction, Stevens-Johnson syndrome, and toxic epidermal necrolysis

	Drug-hypersensitivity syndrome	Serum sickness–like reaction	Stevens-Johnson syndrome, toxic epidermal necrolysis
Symptoms	Fever, cutaneous eruption, internal organ involvement	Fever, cutaneous eruption, arthralgias	Fever, cough, malaise, macular exanthem with mucosal involvement
Laboratory abnormalities	Atypical lymphocytosis with prominent eosinophilia; laboratory abnormalities dependent on the organ involved	Milk leukocytosis with eosinophilia	Leucopenia, occasional liver function test abnormalities
Onset of symptoms	2–8 wk	7–14 d	2–8 wk
Implicated drugs	Aromatic anticonvulsants (phenytoin, phenobarbital, carbamazepine), lamotrigine, allopurinol, dapsone, sulfonamide antibiotics	Beta-lactam antibiotics (especially cefaclor), sulfonamide antibiotics, minocycline	Aromatic anticonvulsants, lamotrigine, sulfonamide antibiotics, allopurinol, dapsone, piroxicam

the reaction in many patients [1]. A generalized exanthem occurs in approximately 85% of patients and usually occurs simultaneously with the appearance of the fever or shortly after. Skin manifestations can range from an exanthematous eruption to more serious eruptions, such as exfoliative dermatitis [5]. Conjunctivitis and angioedema of the face may also be present in some patients [5]. In patients with anticonvulsant-induced hypersensitivity syndrome, facial edema may be present [6]. Liver abnormalities, presenting as elevated transaminases, alkaline phosphatase, prothrombin time, and bilirubin, are present in approximately 50% of patients. In some patients, development of severe hepatitis with jaundice may occur [7]. Other organs, such as the kidney (interstitial nephritis, vasculitis), central nervous system (encephalitis, aseptic meningitis), or the lungs (interstitial pneumonitis, respiratory distress syndrome, vasculitis) may less commonly be involved. A small subgroup of patients may become hypothyroid as part of an autoimmune thyroiditis within 2 months of initiation of symptoms [8]. This is characterized by a low thyroxine level, an elevated level of thyroid-stimulating hormone, and thyroid autoantibodies, including antimicrosomal antibodies. An under-reported toxicity with hypersensitivity syndrome is colitis. This presents with bloody diarrhea and abdominal pain and has led to fatal surgical intervention. The pathology shows a mixed inflammatory infiltrate analogous to the renal histologic changes.

Causative drugs

Anticonvulsants

The hypersensitivity syndrome has been associated with the aromatic anticonvulsants, namely phenytoin, phenobarbital, and carbamazepine [9]. There is evidence that the formation of toxic metabolites by phenytoin, carbamazepine, and phenobarbital may play a pivotal role in the development of hypersensitivity syndrome [10]. Phenytoin, carbamazepine, and phenobarbital are metabolized by various cytochrome P-450 (CYP) enzymes to chemically reactive metabolites, although the specific metabolite is unknown. This metabolite is thought to be detoxified by epoxide hydroxylases. However, if detoxification is defective, the toxic metabolite may act as a hapten and initiate an immunologic response, causing cell necrosis directly or indirectly via pathways leading to apoptosis. Recent work suggests that there is an association between human herpesvirus 6 (HHV-6) infection (either initial infection or reactivation) and severe hypersensitivity syndrome [11,12]. Viral infections may act as, or generate the production of, danger signals leading to damaging immune responses to drugs, rather than immune tolerance [13].

In one study [10], 75% of a series of patients with anticonvulsant hypersensitivity syndrome to one aromatic anticonvulsant showed in vitro cross-reactivity to the other two. In addition, in vitro testing showed that there is a familial occurrence of hypersensitivity to anticonvulsants [10].

Although lamotrigine is not an aromatic anticonvulsant, several reports have documented a hypersensitivity syndrome associated with its use as well [14]. Data demonstrate that a reactive metabolite may also be important in the pathogenesis of lamotrigine hypersensitivity syndrome [15]. Lamotrigine was not seen to cross-react with the other anticonvulsants.

Sulfonamide antibiotics

Sulfonamide antibiotics have also been reported to cause hypersensitivity syndrome in susceptible individuals [16]. The primary metabolic pathway for sulfonamides involves acetylation to a nontoxic metabolite, followed by renal excretion. An alternative metabolic pathway, quantitatively more important in slow acetylators, involves the CYP enzymes [17]. These enzymes can transform the parent compound to reactive metabolites, namely hydroxylamines and nitroso compounds, that produce cytotoxicity independent of a preformed drug-specific antibody [18]. In most individuals, detoxification of the metabolite occurs. However, in patients unable to detoxify this metabolite (eg, glutathione-deficient patients), development of hypersensitivity syndrome may occur [19]. The detoxification defect is present in 2% of the population, but only 1 in 10,000 people manifest symptoms of hypersensitivity syndrome. However, the patient's siblings and other first-degree relatives are at an increased risk (perhaps one in four) of having a similar defect. Other aromatic amines, such as procainamide, dapsone, and acebutolol, are metabolized to similar compounds. Because of the potential for cross-reactivity, clinicians generally recommend avoidance of these drugs in patients who develop symptoms compatible with a sulfonamide hypersensitivity syndrome. However, cross-reactivity with sulfonamides should not occur with related drugs that are not aromatic amines (eg, sulfonylureas, thiazide diuretics, furosemide, and acetazolamide) [20]. Some evidence suggests that, like hypersensitivity syndrome due to anticonvulsants and allopurinol, reactivation of a latent HHV-6 infection may be linked to the development of sulfonamide-induced hypersensitivity syndrome [21].

Dapsone

There are several reports of dapsone-induced hypersensitivity syndrome, also known as the sulfone syndrome [22], in patients treated with this agent for a variety of dermatologic conditions, including leprosy, dermatitis herpetiformis, acne vulgaris, psoriasis, and lupus erythematosus [23]. Dapsone-induced hypersensitivity syndrome usually occurs 4 or more weeks after initiation of therapy and is typified by fever, rash, and hepatitis [22,24].

Dapsone is metabolized primarily via two pathways—N-acetylation and N-hydroxylation. N-acetylation is mediated by N-acetyltransferase type 2, whereas N-hydroxylation is mediated primarily by CYP 3A4. Reactive intermediate metabolites produced by N-hydroxylation, such as hydroxylamines, are formed. These can induce hemolytic anemia and methemoglobinemia. In addition, these reactive metabolites are involved in the pathogenesis of dapsone-induced hypersensitivity syndrome [22]. Cimetidine, an inhibitor of CYP 3A4, has been shown to reduce the formation of the toxic hydroxylamine metabolites of dapsone in vitro, but does not affect acetylation of dapsone [25]. Subsequent studies showed that long-term (at least 3 months) concurrent cimetidine use results in increased plasma dapsone levels, without an increase in hemolysis, and with reduced methemoglobinemia [26]. Whether or not concurrent use of dapsone and cimetidine also reduces the incidence of dapsone hypersensitivity syndrome is unknown.

Minocycline

Hypersensitivity syndrome has also been associated with minocycline [2], usually occurring 2 to 4 weeks after therapy is started. The pathogenesis of minocycline-induced hypersensitivity syndrome is unknown. However, minocycline metabolism may generate an iminoquinone derivative, which is a reactive metabolite. Neither tetracycline nor doxycycline contains the amino acid side chain that has the potential to form a reactive metabolite; this may support the medical experience that neither tetracycline nor doxycycline is associated with hypersensitivity syndrome [27]. However, certainty regarding the absence of cross-reactivity between minocycline and other tetracyclines is lacking. Therefore, caution is advised regarding administration of other tetracyclines in patients who develop a hypersensitivity syndrome after minocycline.

Other drugs

Allopurinol. Allopurinol is associated with the development of serious drug reactions, including hypersensitivity syndrome. In a review of 13 patients with allopurinol adverse reactions, fever and rash were the most common presenting symptoms. Other associated abnormalities included leukocytosis (62%), eosinophilia (54%), renal impairment (54%), and liver dysfunction (69%) [3]. In a patient who developed a hypersensitivity syndrome reaction with hepatitis, reactivation of HHV-6 occurred. HHV-6 DNA in his blood by polymerase chain reaction analysis was positive. As well, HHV-6 DNA in the cerebrospinal fluid was detected [28]. Allopurinol-induced adverse reactions, including hypersensitivity syndrome, Stevens-Johnson syndrome, and toxic epidermal necrolysis, have been strongly associated with a genetic predisposition in Han Chinese. The HLA-B*5801 allele was found to be an important genetic risk factor [29].

Nevirapine. Nevirapine has been associated with hypersensitivity syndrome involving various combinations of fever, hepatitis, or rash. Studies have suggested that HLA-DRB1*0101 and the CD4 status of a patient may determine susceptibility to nevirapine hypersensitivity [30].

Abacavir. Abacavir is also associated with a potentially life-threatening adverse reaction in approximately 8% of patients initiated on this drug. Hypersensitivity syndrome reaction from abacavir has been strongly linked to certain HLA alleles, especially in white populations [31]. Eighteen Caucasian patients from Western Australia with a history of hypersensitivity syndrome were compared with 167 control patients. HLA-B*5701 was overrepresented in patients with hypersensitivity syndrome; it was present in 78% of them and only 2% of controls. The presence of an ancestral haplotype HLA-B*5701, HLA-DR7, and HLA-DQ3 were seen in 72% of patients and in none of the control patients—a positive predictive value of 100% and a negative predictive value of 97%. In a North American post-abacavir hypersensitivity population, the frequency of HLA-B*5701 was 55%. None of the African-American patients in the study possessed the allele [32]. Further studies are needed before genetic testing can be relied upon to help, for example, in the decision to rechallenge a patient with abacavir.

Differential diagnosis

The differential diagnosis of hypersensitivity syndrome includes other cutaneous drug reactions, acute viral infections (eg, Epstein-Barr virus, hepatitis virus, influenza virus, cytomegalovirus), lymphoma, and idiopathic hypereosinophilic syndrome. After hypersensitivity syndrome has been recognized by the symptom complex of fever, rash, and lymphadenopathy, a minimum number of laboratory tests help to evaluate internal organ involvement, which may be asymptomatic. Liver transaminases, complete blood count, urinalysis, and serum creatinine should be performed at the initial evaluation. In addition, the clinician should be guided by the presence of symptoms, which may suggest specific internal organ involvement (eg, respiratory symptoms). Thyroid function tests should be measured and repeated in 2 to 3 months. A skin biopsy may be helpful if the patient has a blistering or a pustular eruption. Unfortunately, there are no readily available diagnostic or confirmatory tests to establish drug causation. An in vitro test using a mouse hepatic microsomal system is used for research purposes to evaluate patients who develop hypersensitivity syndrome [33]. Oral rechallenges are not recommended due to the severity of the hypersensitivity syndrome reactions. Patch testing has been helpful in some cases of anticonvulsant hypersensitivity syndrome and betalactam-induced hypersensitivity syndrome in the authors' clinic. Patch testing for abacavir hypersensitivity syndrome has shown promise and large clinical trials to confirm the role of patch testing are underway [34].

Management

Although the role of systemic corticosteroid therapy is controversial, most clinicians would elect to start prednisone at a dose of 1 to 2 mg/kg/d if symptoms are severe. In contrast to the issue of corticosteroids in Stevens-Johnson syndrome and toxic epidermal necrolysis, there is no significant barrier function alteration (ie, skin sloughing) leading to the potential for sepsis in the hypersensitivity syndrome. There are cases of patients who have been treated with cyclosporine [35] or intravenous immunoglobulin [36]. Antihistamines or topical corticosteroids can also be used to alleviate symptoms. Because the risk of hypersensitivity syndrome is substantially increased in first-degree relatives of patients who had hypersensitivity syndrome reactions, counseling of family members is a crucial part of the assessment of this syndrome [10].

Serum sickness and serum sickness–like reactions

Serum sickness is a clinical syndrome characterized by fever, lymphadenopathy, arthralgias, cutaneous eruptions, gastrointestinal disturbances, and malaise and is often associated with proteinuria, without evidence of glomerulonephritis [37]. It was first described with the injection of foreign proteins, such as equine antitoxins, snake and spider antivenins, antilymphocyte globulins, and streptokinase. Serum sickness is mediated by the tissue deposition of circulating immune complexes, the activation of complement, and the ensuing inflammatory response.

In contrast, serum sickness–like reactions (SSLRs) are defined by the presence of fever, rash (usually urticarial), and arthralgias occurring 1 to 3 weeks after drug initiation [38]. Other findings, such as lymphadenopathy and eosinophilia, may also be present. However, immune complexes, hypocomplementemia, vasculitis, and renal lesions are absent in SSLRs.

Epidemiologic studies in children suggest that the risk of SSLRs is greater with cefaclor as compared with other antibiotic therapy, including other cephalosporins [39]. The overall incidence rate of cefaclor SSLR has been estimated to be approximately 0.024% to 0.2% per course of cefaclor prescribed. Although the pathogenesis is unknown, it has been postulated that in genetically susceptible hosts, a reactive cefaclor metabolite is generated during its metabolism that may bind with tissue proteins and elicit an inflammatory response manifesting as SSLR [40].

Other drugs that have recently been implicated in the causation of SSLRs include minocycline [2], bupropion [41], and rituximab [42,43]. The incidence rates for these drugs are unknown.

Management

Discontinuation of the culprit drug and symptomatic treatment with antihistamines and topical corticosteroids are recommended in patients with SSLR. A short course of oral corticosteroids may be required in patients with more severe symptoms [38]. The drug causing the SSLR should be avoided in the future. For cefaclor and cefprozil, the risk of cross-reaction with other beta-lactam antibiotics is small and the further administration of another cephalosporin is usually well tolerated [44]. However, some clinicians recommend that patients who experience serum sickness–like reactions from cefaclor avoid all beta-lactam drugs. No information is available regarding cross-reactivity among the tetracycline antibiotics in patients with minocycline SSLR.

Acute generalized exanthematous pustulosis

AGEP is characterized by a fever above 38°C and a cutaneous eruption with nonfollicular sterile pustules on an edematous erythematous background. The interval between drug administration and the onset of the eruption can vary from 2 days to 3 weeks. A long interval probably indicates primary sensitization and the shorter interval may be related to an unintentional reexposure [45]. The onset is usually abrupt, with the eruption starting on the face and spreading to the trunk and lower limbs. Two weeks later, generalized desquamation occurs. Some patients may present with additional skin lesions, including petechial purpura, erythema multiforme–like target lesions, vesicles, or blisters [46]. Characteristic laboratory findings include leukocytosis, which is usually neutrophilic. The spongiform pustule is the major histologic feature of AGEP; papillary dermal edema, polymorphous perivascular infiltrates with eosinophils, leukocytoclastic vasculitis, and necrotic keratinocytes may also be evident [46].

AGEP is most commonly associated with anti-infective agents, including beta-lactam and macrolide antibiotics and terbinafine [45,47]. However, many other drugs have been implicated, including herbal medications, gefitinib, calcium channel blockers, and analgesics [48,49]. Differential diagnosis includes pustular psoriasis, hypersensitivity syndrome with pustulation, and Sneddon-Wilkinson disease [45].

Discontinuation of therapy is usually the extent of treatment necessary in most patients. However, the use of systemic corticosteroids may be indicated in some patients, depending on the extent of the reaction. Re-administration (rechallenge) of the suspected drug is not recommended because recurrence of lesions usually occurs within hours of drug administration [50].

Patch testing has been used to aid in the diagnosis of AGEP [51], usually producing an isomorphic pustular reaction with subcorneal pustules on the biopsy specimen. The tests are often positive within 6 hours [50]. Positive patch tests and lymphocyte transformation tests suggest involvement of T cells in AGEP. Drug-specific CD4+ and CD8+ T cells have been isolated from patch test sites and blood from patients with a history of AGEP [52].

Drug-induced linear IgA disease

Linear IgA disease is an autoimmune bullous dermatosis that is identified on the basis of the linear deposition of IgA at the basement membrane zone [53]. This disease can be induced by such drugs as vancomycin, lithium, diclofenac, and amiodarone. Drug-induced linear IgA disease usually develops within 1 to 15 days of the first dose of the inducing medication and resolves within 2 weeks of discontinuation [54]. The drug-induced disease probably represents an immunologic response to the offending drug.

Drug-induced linear IgA disease is heterogeneous in clinical presentation. Cases have shown morphologies resembling erythema multiforme, bullous pemphigoid, and dermatitis herpetiformis. Mucosal involvement occurs in approximately 40% to 45% of cases of drug-induced linear IgA disease. Drug-induced disease cannot be distinguished from the idiopathic variety either clinically, histologically, or immunologically. However, the clinical courses of these presentations differ. In drug-induced disease, spontaneous remission occurs once the offending agent is withdrawn; in idiopathic linear IgA disease, immune deposits disappear from the skin once the lesions resolve. Systemic corticosteroids and dapsone do not influence the healing process in drug-induced disease, whereas these agents have been proven effective in treatment of idiopathic linear IgA disease [55].

Stevens-Johnson syndrome and toxic epidermal necrolysis

The spectrum of severe cutaneous adverse reactions, which may represent variants of the same disease process, includes Stevens-Johnson syndrome and toxic epidermal necrolysis. Erythema multiforme (EM), EM major, and atypical EM major are cutaneous reactions that are usually seen postinfection rather than postdrug. Severe cases of EM major and atypical EM major can be confused with Stevens-Johnson syndrome. Most investigators believe that Stevens-Johnson syndrome and toxic epidermal necrolysis are on a spectrum of severity and are different than the EM diseases.

The incidence of toxic epidermal necrolysis in adults secondary to sulfamethoxazole-trimethoprim was found to be 2.6 per 100,000 exposures. However, in HIV-positive patients, the rate was 8.4 cases per 100,000 exposures [56]. A prodromal phase of fever, cough, and malaise is followed by a macular exanthem, which progresses to become Nikolsky positive. In patients with toxic epidermal necrolysis, the gastrointestinal tract can be involved, and up to 30% of cases may have respiratory involvement. In addition, abnormalities in liver function tests have been reported. Significant leucopenia is a common finding as well [57].

Differentiation among cases of Stevens-Johnson syndrome and toxic epidermal necrolysis depends on the nature of the skin lesions and extent of body surface area involvement. The more severe forms of toxic epidermal necrolysis have a greater percentage of body surface area of epidermal detachment. Target lesions tend to change from the classic, raised, three-ringed iris lesion to a more purpuric or erythematous two-ringed lesion. Clinically, each of these reaction patterns is characterized by the presence of the triad of mucous membrane erosions, target lesions, and epidermal necrosis with skin detachment [58]. Some Stevens-Johnson syndrome cases are not drug related and may develop after a variety of other predisposing factors, including infections (eg, mycoplasma-induced pneumonia), neoplasia, and autoimmune diseases. The most frequent drugs cited as causes for Stevens-Johnson syndrome and toxic epidermal necrolysis are the anticonvulsants, sulfonamide antibiotics, nonsteroidal anti-inflammatory drugs (especially piroxicam), and allopurinol [59].

The pathogenesis of Stevens-Johnson syndrome and toxic epidermal necrolysis is unknown, although a metabolic basis has been hypothesized [10,60]. Sulfonamides and anticonvulsants, which are the two groups of drugs most frequently associated with Stevens-Johnson syndrome and toxic epidermal necrolysis, are metabolized to toxic metabolites that are subsequently detoxified in most individuals. However, in predisposed patients with a genetic defect, the metabolite may bind covalently to proteins. In some of these patients, the metabolite-protein adducts may trigger an immune response that may lead to cutaneous adverse drug reactions. Some evidence supports the role for the "cell death" receptor Fas and its ligand FasL in the pathogenesis of keratinocyte apopotosis during toxic epidermal necrolysis [61]. In addition, activated T cells, macrophages, and neutrophils may be triggers for the development of toxic epidermal necrolysis [62]. Drug-specific major histocompatibility complex class I-restricted, perforin- and granzyme-mediated cytotoxicity may have a primary role in the development of toxic epidermal necrolysis [63]. A recent study in a Han Chinese population has shown that HLA-B*1502 may act as a genetic marker for carbamazepine-induced Stevens-Johnson syndrome, with an odds ratio that was >2504:1 [64].

Management

To rule out concurrent internal organ involvement, complete blood counts, liver enzymes, and chest radiographs should be performed. Increasing age, significant comorbidity, and a greater extent of skin involvement correlate with a worse prognosis [65]. Treatment of Stevens-Johnson syndrome and toxic epidermal necrolysis includes discontinuation of a suspected drug and provision of supportive measures, such as careful wound care, hydration, ophthalmologic assessment, and nutritional support. Ocular complications are not infrequent and have a significant impact on long-term morbidity. In one study, 79% of patients with ocular involvement in the acute phase of toxic epidermal necrolysis had long-term ocular complications [66].

The use of systemic corticosteroids in Stevens-Johnson syndrome and toxic epidermal necrolysis is controversial. Some clinicians believe corticosteroids may be beneficial when administered early in the disease and at relatively high dosage. However, other investigators suggest that corticosteroids do not shorten the recovery time and may increase the risk of complications, including secondary infections (potentially leading to sepsis) and gastrointestinal bleeding [59]. Most clinicians avoid systemic corticosteroids, especially in severe cases [57,60]. Uncontrolled studies showed that plasmapheresis [67] and cyclosporine [57,68] may be beneficial. Some centers use high-dose human intravenous immunoglobulin [69]. There have been numerous case reports and noncontrolled clinical studies that have investigated the effects of intravenous immunoglobulin in patients with Stevens-Johnson syndrome or toxic epidermal necrolysis [70]. Six of the eight studies suggest a benefit of intravenous immunoglobulin at doses greater than 2 g/kg on the mortality associated with toxic epidermal necrolysis [61]. However, other studies have not found an improved outcome in patients with toxic epidermal necrolysis who are treated with intravenous immunoglobulin [71]. Patients who have developed a severe cutaneous adverse reaction (eg, Stevens-Johnson syndrome or toxic epidermal necrolysis) should not be rechallenged with the suspected causative drug nor should they undergo desensitization with the medication.

Summary

Because severe reactions in the skin are debilitating and potentially lethal, offending drugs are quickly withdrawn. Because reactions are rare, it has been difficult to develop clear clinical guidelines in management. Clinicians must maintain a high index of suspicion regarding the possibility of drug-induced disorders, must be aware of the clues for accurate diagnosis, and must treat the individual based on evidence as well as on the patient's specific needs. Careful clinical and laboratory assessment is warranted, including evaluations for possible internal organ involvement, especially with reactions such as hypersensitivity syndrome, Stevens-Johnson syndrome, and toxic epidermal necrolysis.

References

[1] Roujeau JC, Stern R. Severe adverse cutaneous reactions to drugs. N Engl J Med 1994;331:1272–85.

[2] Knowles S, Shapiro L, Shear N. Serious adverse reactions induced by minocycline: a report of 13 patients and review of the literature. Arch Dermatol 1996;132:934–9.

[3] Khoo B, Leow Y. A review of inpatients with adverse drug reactions to allopurinol. Singapore Med J 2000;41:156–60.

[4] Tennis P, Stern R. Risk of serious cutaneous disorders after initiation of use of phenytoin, carbamazepine, or sodium valproate: a record linkage study. Neurology 1997;49:542–6.

[5] Baba M, Karakas M, Aksungur V, et al. The anticonvulsant hypersensitivity syndrome. J Eur Acad Dermatol Venereol 2003;17:399–401.

[6] Choi T, Doh K, Kim S, et al. Clinicopathological and genotypic aspects of anticonvulsant-induced pseudolymphoma syndrome. Br J Dermatol 2003; 148:730–6.

[7] Knowles S, Shapiro L, Shear N. Anticonvulsant hypersensitivity syndrome: incidence, prevention and management. Drug Saf 1999;21:489–501.

[8] Gupta A, Eggo M, Uetrecht J, et al. Drug-induced hypothyroidism: the thyroid as a target organ in hypersensitivity reactions to anticonvulsants and sulfonamides. Clin Pharmacol Ther 1992;51:56–67.

[9] Vittorio C, Muglia J. Anticonvulsant hypersensitivity syndrome. Arch Intern Med 1995;155:2285–90.

[10] Shear N, Spielberg S. Anticonvulsant hypersensitivity syndrome, in vitro assessment of risk. J Clin Invest 1988;82:1826–32.

[11] Descamps V, Valance A, Edlinger C, et al. Association of human herpesvirus 6 infection with drug reaction with eosinophilia and systemic symptoms. Arch Dermatol 2001;137:301–4.

[12] Kano Y, Inaoka M, Shiohara T. Association between anticonvulsant hypersensitivity syndrome and human herpesvirus 6 reactivation and hypogammaglobulinemia. Arch Dermatol 2004;140:183–8.

[13] Wong G, Shear N. Is a drug alone sufficient to cause the drug hypersensitivity syndrome? Arch Dermatol 2004;140:226–30.

[14] Schlienger R, Knowles S, Shear N. Lamotrigine-associated anticonvulsant hypersensitivity syndrome. Neurology 1998;51:1172–5.

[15] Sullivan JR, Neuman M, Knowles S, et al. Evidence for reactive drug metabolites in lamotrigine-associated drug hypersensitivity syndrome. J Cut Med Surg 2000;4:38.

[16] Epstein M, Wright J. Severe multisystem disease caused by trimethoprim-sulfamethoxazole: possible role of an in vitro lymphocyte assay. J Allergy Clin Immunol 1990;86:416–7.

[17] Ohtani T, Hiroi A, Sakurane M, et al. Slow acetylator genotypes as a possible risk factor for infectious mononucleosis-like syndrome induced by salazosulfapyridine. Br J Dermatol 2003;148:1035–9.

[18] Cribb A, Spielberg S. Sulfamethoxazole is metabolized to the hydroxylamine in humans. Clin Pharmacol Ther 1992;51:522–6.

[19] Shear N, Spielberg S, Grant D, et al. Differences in metabolism of sulfonamides predisposing to idiosyncratic toxicity. Ann Intern Med 1986;105:179–84.

[20] Knowles S, Shapiro L, Shear N. Should celecoxib be contraindicated in patients who are allergic to sulfonamides? Revisiting the meaning of "sulfa" allergy. Drug Saf 2001;24:239–47.

[21] Morimoto T, Sato T, Matsuoka A, et al. Trimethoprim-sulfamethoxazole-induced hypersensitivity syndrome associated with reactivation of human herpesvirus-6. Intern Med 2006;45:101–5.

[22] Prussick R, Shear NH. Dapsone hypersensitivity syndrome. J Am Acad Dermatol 1996;35:346–9.

[23] Sener O, Doganci L, Safali M, et al. Severe dapsone hypersensitivity syndrome. J Investig Allergol Clin Immunol 2006;16:268–70.

[24] Agrawal S, Agarwalla A. Dapsone hypersensitivity syndrome: a clinico-epidemiological review. J Dermatolog Treat 2005;32:883–9.

[25] Coleman M, Scott A, Breckenridge A, et al. The use of cimetidine as a selective inhibitor of dapsone N-hydroxylation in man. Br J Clin Pharmacol 1990; 30:761–7.

[26] Rhodes L, Tingle M, Park B, et al. Cimetidine improves the therapeutic/toxic ratio of dapsone in patients on chronic dapsone therapy. Br J Dermatol 1995;132:257–62.

[27] Shapiro L, Knowles S, Shear N. Comparative safety and risk management of tetracycline, doxycline and minocycline. Arch Dermatol 1997;133:1224–30.

[28] Masaki T, Fukunaga A, Tohyama M, et al. Human herpes virus 6 encephalitis in allopurinol-induced hypersensitivity syndrome. Acta Derm Venereol 2003;83:128–31.

[29] Hung S, Chung W, Liou L, et al. HLA-B*5801 allele as a genetic marker for severe cutaneous adverse reactions caused by allopurinol. Proc Natl Acad Sci U S A 2005;102:4134–9.

[30] Martin A, Nolan D, James I, et al. Predisposition to nevirapine hypersensitivity associated with HLA-DRB1*0101 and abrogated by low CD4 T-cell counts. AIDS 2005;19:97–9.

[31] Mallal S, Nolan D, Witt C, et al. Association between the presence of HLAB5701, HLADR7 and HLA-DQ3 and hypersensitivity to HIV-1 reverse transcriptase inhibitor abacavir. Lancet 2002;359:727–32.

[32] Hetherington S, Hughes A, Mosteller M, et al. Genetic variations in HLA-B region and hypersensitivity reactions to abacavir. Lancet 2002;359:1121–2.

[33] Neuman M, Malkiewicz I, Shear N. A novel lymphocyte toxicity assay to assess drug hypersensitivity syndromes. Clin Biochem 2000;33:517–24.

[34] Phillips E, Wong G, Kaul R, et al. Clinical and immunogenetic correlates of abacavir hypersensitivity. AIDS 2005;19:979–81.

[35] Harman K, Morris S, Higgins E. Persistent anticonvulsant hypersensitivity syndrome responding to ciclosporin. Clin Exp Dermatol 2003;28:364–5.

[36] Kano Y, Inaoka M, Sakuma K, et al. Virus reactivation and intravenous immunoglobulin (IVIG) therapy of drug-induced hypersensitivity syndromes. Toxicology 2005;209:165–7.

[37] Lawley T, Bielory L, Gascon P, et al. A prospective clinical and immunologic analysis of patients with serum sickness. N Engl J Med 1984;311:1407–13.

[38] King B, Geelhoed G. Adverse skin and joint reactions associated with oral antibiotics in children: the role of cefaclor in serum sickness-like reactions. J Paediatr Child Health 2003;39:677–81.

[39] Heckbert S, Stryker W, Coltin K, et al. Serum sickness in children after antibiotic exposure: estimates of occurence and morbidity in a Health Maintenance Organization population. Am J Epidemiol 1990;132: 336–42.

[40] Kearns G, Wheeler J, Childress S, et al. Serum sickness-like reactions to cefaclor: role of hepatic metabolism and individual susceptibility. J Pediatr 1994; 125:805–11.

[41] McCollom R, Elbe D, Ritchie A. Bupropion-induced serum sickness-like reaction. Ann Pharmacother 2000;34:471–3.

[42] Herishanu Y. Rituximab-induced serum sickness. Am J Hematol 2002;70:329.

[43] Schutgens R. Rituximab-induced serum sickness. Br J Haematol 2006;135:147.

[44] Reynolds R. Cefaclor and serum sickness-like reaction. JAMA 1996;276:950–1.

[45] Beltraminelli H, Lerch M, Arnold A, et al. Acute generalized exanthematous pustulosis induced by the antifungal terbinafine: case report and review of the literature. Br J Dermatol 2005;152:780–3.

[46] Sidoroff A, Haleevy S, Bainck J, et al. Acute generalized exanthematous pustulosis (AGEP):

a clinical reaction pattern. J Cutan Pathol 2001;28: 113–9.

[47] Roujeau J, Bioulac-Sage P, Bourseau C, et al. Acute generalized exanthematous pustulosis: analysis of 63 cases. Arch Dermatol 1991;127:1333–8.

[48] Manzur A, Kiyani K. Acute generalized exanthematous pustulosis triggered by intake of herbal medications. Int J Dermatol 2006;45:1247–8.

[49] Shih H, Hsiao Y, Wu M, et al. Gefitinib-induced acute generalized exanthematous pustulosis in two patients with advanced non-small-cell lung cancer. Br J Dermatol 2006;155:1101–2.

[50] Beylot C, Doutre M, Beylot-Barry M. Acute generalized exanthematous pustulosis. Semin Cutan Med Surg 1996;15:244–9.

[51] Barbaud A. Drug patch testing in systemic cutaneous drug allergy. Toxicology 2005;209:209–16.

[52] Britschgi M, Pichler W. Acute generalized exanthematous pustulosis, a clue to neturphil-mediated inflammatory processes orchestrated by T cells. Curr Opin Allergy Clin Immunol 2002;2:325–31.

[53] Kuechle M, Stegemeir E, Maynard B, et al. Drug-induced linear IgA bullous dermatosis: report of six cases and review of the literature. J Am Acad Dermatol 1994;30:187–92.

[54] Navi D, Michael D, Fazel N. Drug-induced linear IgA bullous dermatosis. Dermatol Online J 2006;12:12.

[55] Neughebauer B, Negron G, Pelton S, et al. Bullous skin disease: an unusual allergic reaction to vancomycin. Am J Med Sci 2002;323:273–8.

[56] Gimnig J, MacArthur J, M'bang'ombe M, et al. Severe cutaneous reactions to sulfadoxine-pyramethamine and trimethoprim-sulfamethoxazole in Blantyre District, Malawi. Am J Trop Med Hyg 2006;74:738–43.

[57] Chave T, Mortimer N, Sladden M, et al. Toxic epidermal necrolysis: current evidence, practical management and future directions. Br J Dermatol 2005;153:241–53.

[58] Bastuji-Garin S, Rzany B, Stern R, et al. Clinical classification of cases of toxic epidermal necrolysis, Stevens-Johnson syndrome, and erythema multiforme. Arch Dermatol 1993;129:92–6.

[59] Wolf R, Orion E, Marcos B, et al. Life-threatening acute adverse cutaneous drug reactions. Clin Dermatol 2005;23:171–81.

[60] Bachot N, Roujeau J. Physiopathology and treatment of severe drug eruptions. Curr Opin Allergy Clin Immunol 2001;1:293–8.

[61] French L, Trent J, Kerdel F. Use of intravenous immunoglobulin in toxic epidermal necrolysis and Stevens-Johnson syndrome: our current understanding. Int Immunopharmacol 2006;6: 543–9.

[62] Caproni M, Torchia D, Schincaglia E, et al. The CD40/CD40 ligand system is expressed in the cutaneous lesions of erythema multiforme and Stevens-Johnson syndrome/toxic epidermal necrolysis spectrum. Br J Dermatol 2006;154:319–24.

[63] Nassif A, Bensussan A, Boumsell L, et al. Toxic epidermal necrolysis: effector cells are drug-specific cytotoxic T cells. J Allergy Clin Immunol 2004;114: 1209–15.

[64] Chung W, Hung S, Hong H, et al. Medical genetics: a marker for Stevens-Johnson syndrome. Nature 2004;428:486.

[65] Ducic I, Shalom A, Rising W, et al. Outcome of patients with toxic epidermal necrolysis syndrome revisited. Plast Reconstr Surg 2002;110:768–73.

[66] Oplatek A, Brown K, Sen S, et al. Long-term follow-up of patients treated for toxic epidermal necrolysis. J Burn Care Res 2006;27:26–33.

[67] Cahdemenos GC, Chrysamallis F, Sambolos K, et al. Plasmapheresis in toxic epidermal necrolysis. Int J Dermatol 1997;36:218–21.

[68] Arevalo J, Lorente J, Gonzalez-Herrada C, et al. Treatment of toxic epidermal necrolysis with cyclosporin A. J Trauma 2000;48:473–8.

[69] Prins C, kerdel F, Padilla R, et al. Treatment of toxic epidermal necrolysis with high-dose intravenous immunoglobulins: multicenter retrospective analysis of 48 consecutive cases. Arch Dermatol 2003;139: 26–32.

[70] Mittmann N, Chan B, Knowles S, et al. Intravenous immunoglobulin use in patients with toxic epidermal necrolysis and Stevens-Johnson syndrome. Am J Clin Dermatol 2006;7:359–68.

[71] Shortt R, Gomez M, Mittmann N, et al. Intravenous immunoglobulin does not improve outcome in toxic epidermal necrolysis. J Burn Care Rehabil 2004;25: 246–55.

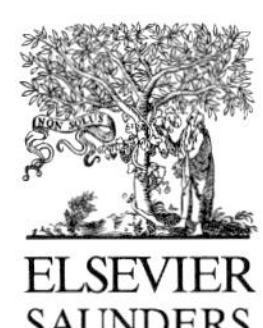

ELSEVIER
SAUNDERS

Dermatol Clin 25 (2007) 255–261

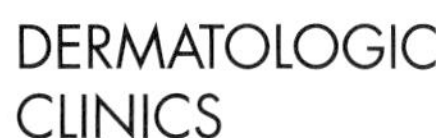

Newly Recognized Cutaneous Drug Eruptions

Jeffrey P. Callen, MD

Division of Dermatology, University of Louisville School of Medicine, Louisville, KY 40292, USA

As innovation in medicine occurs and new drugs are developed, there is a potential for the occurrence of an increasing number of cutaneous drug reactions. There are many new medications for the treatment of systemic disease as well as for the treatment of skin disease. Every such advance is associated with potential adverse reactions including skin eruptions. In some instances cutaneous disease is anticipated during drug development, whereas in other cases the cutaneous disease is one of the rare manifestations that is noted in postmarketing use of the agent.

Innovation comes at a potential cost to the humans who volunteer for studies of new therapies. Witness the recent article in the *New England Journal of Medicine* on cytokine storm that occurred with a presumably sterile agent (TGN1412), which is a superagonistic humanized monoclonal antibody designed to stimulate and expand T-cell populations independent of the T-cell receptor [1]. In this instance, there were eight volunteers who were given an infusion of the agent of whom six became acutely ill with multiorgan failure including disseminated intravascular coagulopathy. In all of the patients a prominent generalized erythema was part of the process and in at least two individuals severe desquamation complicated the late stage of the reaction. There was no mention of mucosal abnormalities or blistering. More than likely, unless a contaminant is found, this agent will not proceed in its development.

In the accompanying editorial comment, Drazen [2] stated,

> "It is certainly possible to change the way in which novel agents are tested to minimize the number of subjects who are put at risk. As long

as we continue to manipulate biology in new ways, we probably cannot prevent all such events from occurring. We must do what we can to minimize risk, but the future health of the world population demands that we not let adverse events put an end to medical progress. We must treat those at risk with respect and great care, but the work must go on. The troubling fact of the matter is that without people who are willing to place themselves at risk to advance our knowledge, we will be frozen in our current state of understanding. And this state simply may not be good enough to enable us to meet the next unexpected challenge that comes our way."

This article examines drugs that have made it through the process of development and are on the market for various conditions. In some instances the reactions were predictable, but in others the reactions are idiosyncratic, rare, and were only noted after a large experience with the agent. This article focuses on the following agents and/or eruptions: epidermal growth factor receptor (EGF-R) inhibitors, tyrosine kinase inhibitors, tumor necrosis factor-alpha (TNF-α) antagonists, sildenafil and related compounds, sirolimus, drug-induced cutaneous lupus erythematosus, and the hand-foot syndrome. Some of these agents and issues were discussed in a recent review [3].

Epidermal growth factor receptor inhibitors

There have been articles that have appeared almost monthly on the occurrence of eruptions related to the use of this category of drugs [4–9]. There are three currently approved agents in this class: cetuximab, erlotinib, and gefitinib. In addition, there are multiple other agents that are being studied and will probably come to market in the near future. These agents offer hope to patients with solid tumors that have epidermal growth

---

E-mail address: jefca@aol.com

0733-8635/07/$ - see front matter © 2007 Elsevier Inc. All rights reserved.
doi:10.1016/j.det.2007.01.003

factor receptors on their surface. Two types of agents comprise this class: those that are monoclonal antibodies that bind to the receptor on the surface of cells and down-regulate their expression or cause apoptosis of the cells, and those that are small receptor tyrosine kinase inhibitors that competitively block receptor phosphorylation [6]. Agero and colleagues [6] recently detailed the agents that are under study and divided these two classes of agents into several subsets. The monoclonal antibodies can be fully human (ABX-EGF aka panitumumab), chimeric (Cetuximab), or humanized (EMD 72,000 aka matuzumab or h-R3 aka nimutozumab or cimazumab). The small receptor tyrosine kinase inhibitors can be associated with reversible binding (gefitinib, erlotinib, GW2016 aka iapatinib, or PKI 166) or associated with irreversible binding (EKB-569 or CI-1033 aka canertinib). Cetuximab (Erbitux) is approved for the treatment of metastatic colorectal carcinoma and unresectable squamous cell carcinoma of the head and neck. It is administered intravenously. Gefitinib (Iressa) and erlotinib (Tarceva) are administered orally and are approved for non–small cell carcinoma of the lung. Other indications are likely to be approved in the near future.

Mucocutaneous reactions to these agents include a folliculocentric pustular eruption that has been characterized as acneiform, paronychia and fissuring of the lateral nailfolds and distal fingertips, hair changes, diffuse xerosis, urticaria, and a mucositis. All of the reactions appear to be worse with increasing doses of the drugs with the exception of urticaria and anaphylaxis that is probably idiosyncratic. In addition, it has been observed in multiple reports and studies that the presence of eruptions is associated with a survival advantage and the severity of the eruption also correlates with improved chance of therapeutic response and ultimately, survival.

The mechanism of the folliculocentric eruption is not understood, but EGF-R may be involved in the normal proliferation of keratinocytes and inhibition of these receptors might alter the follicular epithelium. There has been little written about the mechanism of the other skin-related toxicities, and they have not been correlated with survival advantage.

There is no specific management strategy for the eruption associated with EGF-R inhibitors. Cleansers, topical antibiotics, systemic antibiotics, topical retinoids, topical corticosteroids, and calcineurin inhibitors have all been suggested in individual patients [3,6]. In severe reactions, oral corticosteroids or isotretinoin have been proposed for use.

Tyrosine kinase inhibitors

Imatinib (Gleevec) is an oral agent that is approved for first-line therapy of Philadelphia chromosome–positive chronic myelogenous leukemia. The basis of its therapeutic activity is that tyrosine kinase (BCR-ABL) is produced and serves a critical pathogenetic role in the occurrence of chronic myelogenous leukemia. Imatinib also inhibits KIT, which is the product of c-kit and platelet-derived growth factor receptor. This agent is therefore useful for patients with mast cell disease, hypereosinophilic syndrome, metastatic dermatofibrosarcoma protuberans, and chronic myeloproliferative diseases [10].

A variety of eruptions have been reported with imatinib including exanthems, Stevens-Johnson syndrome, exfoliative erythroderma, acute generalized exanthematous pustulosis, lichen planus–like eruptions, pityriasis rosea–like eruptions, neutrophilic dermatoses, and color changes of the hair [3]. Up to half of the patients treated with imatinib are reported to develop some form of cutaneous toxicity, most with exanthems or cutaneous edema. The mechanism of the eruptions is not understood.

As with the EGF-R inhibitors, the skin eruption and edema associated with imatinib appears to be dose related. Unlike the former group of agents, the occurrence of the eruption is not associated with improved responsiveness to the agent or with improved survival.

The more severe reactions, the pityriasis rosea–like eruption [10] and the lichenoid eruption [11] are idiosyncratic and occur in a small minority of patients. Recently an eruption resembling acute febrile neutrophilic dermatosis (Sweet's syndrome) has been described in a patient with chronic myelogenous leukemia treated with imatinib [12]. This eruption has been observed in patients with myelogenous leukemia, but in the reported patient the eruption cleared when the imatinib was stopped and recurred with re-introduction of the drug, thereby linking the occurrence to the drug rather than the underlying disease.

Dasatinib is a second-line tyrosine kinase inhibitor that is also used for similar indications as imatinib. A recent report detailed the development of panniculitis in two patients treated with this agent who were imatinib-resistant [13]. Both patients had chronic myelogenous leukemia and developed fever and tender subcutaneous nodules. Biopsy of the eruption revealed a neutrophilic lobular panniculitis. Cessation of the dasatinib resulted in a resolution of the panniculitis and relapse occurred with rechallenge. Although this could represent a Sweet's panniculitis that could also be associated with chronic myelogenous leukemia, the fact that there was a dechallenge and a rechallenge leads one to the conclusion that the process was indeed drug-related.

Tumor necrosis factor-alpha antagonists

Injection site reactions are the most common side effect for both etanercept and adalimumab, but in general they are of minimal clinical significance [14]. Most are mild to moderate and diminish in frequency after the first month of treatment. Erythema, pruritus, pain, and swelling have been described.

Recent reports of new-onset psoriasis have appeared primarily in patients with rheumatoid arthritis and Crohn's disease [15–18]. The eruption appears to be different from usual forms of psoriasis in that most of the patients have manifest palmoplantar pustular disease. In addition, the eruption frequently occurs after a prolonged course of anti-TNF therapy has been used. de Gannes and colleagues [16] reported one of the largest series of patients with "new-onset" psoriasis, which included patients with rheumatologic diseases such as rheumatoid arthritis (13), psoriatic arthritis (1), and seronegative arthritis (1). The disease was manifest as new-onset disease in 13 patients and as a worsening of psoriasis in 2 patients. All three of the existing TNF antagonists were reported to be linked to their observations. In addition, they examined the immunohistochemical staining of lesional skin in their patients and found staining for anti-myxovirus-resistance protein A, which is a surrogate marker of increased interferon activity. They also examined patients with psoriasis vulgaris and failed to note a similar staining pattern. Withdrawal of the TNF antagonist usually results in improvement of the eruption; however, it is possible in some patients to re-introduce the TNF antagonist or to substitute one of the agents for another and not have a reappearance of the disease. Although the exact mechanism behind this observation is unknown, Fiorentino [19] in an accompanying editorial, suggests that these observations might be the result of an imbalance between TNF-α and

interferon-α and in such instances other external stimuli might allow patients to develop or flare disease that was otherwise quiescent.

Leukocytoclastic vasculitis might complicate therapy with TNF agents [14]. The onset of the disease is often delayed and most of the patients have had underlying rheumatoid arthritis, a disease known to be associated with vasculitis. Cessation of therapy has been associated with improvement of the vasculitis in most patients. I am unaware of any rechallenges with the "offending" agent or another TNF antagonist that have been reported. This occurrence does appear to be quite uncommon and it has been limited to the rheumatoid arthritis population thus far. The mechanism behind this adverse reaction is not known and thus far has not been studied.

An increase in antinuclear antibodies seems to occur irregularly with etanercept. There is one small case series of patients who developed signs and symptoms of systemic lupus erythematosus (SLE), including some who developed skin lesions, while receiving etanercept [20]. Etanercept-induced lupus erythematosus (LE) is readily reversible upon cessation of the drug [21,22]. Despite the observations that etanercept might induce LE-like disease, there are several cases in which the use of etanercept was associated with disappearance of subacute cutaneous lupus erythematosus (SCLE). It is not necessary to evaluate patients for antinuclear antibodies or other serologic tests before or during therapy with etanercept.

Multiple cases of interstitial granulomatous dermatitis have been reported in patients on various anti-TNF agents [14]. Last, there are reports of several patients who developed an eosinophilic cellulitis while on etanercept or adalimumab [23,24].

Sildenafil and related compounds

Sildenafil is a phosphodiesterase type-5 inhibitor that is indicated for treatment of erectile dysfunction. There are a large number of patients who take this or a related agent intermittently on a chronic basis. One patient developed a lichenoid eruption while taking this agent and following withdrawal for 3 weeks the eruption resolved. Four weeks later sildenafil was reintroduced and the eruption re-appeared [25]. Another patient was reported to develop toxic epidermal necrolysis following the ingestion of sildenafil [26]; however, in this case report the patient had also ingested an aphrodisiac Chinese herbal medicine around the same time, so it is not clear if sildenafil was the cause.

Sirolimus

Sirolimus is a product of *Streptomyces hygroscopisus* that is used for prevention of allograft rejection. It can be used as a primary therapy or as a therapy for patients who have had toxicity from calcineurin inhibitors. This agent has been associated with frequent cutaneous adverse reactions, particularly acne-like eruptions. Mahé and colleagues [27,28] in two separate reports noted that acne occurs in roughly 45% of patients treated with sirolimus. They noted that the onset was relatively soon after the introduction of the therapy. Importantly, the disease differs from acne vulgaris in that only inflammatory lesions (primarily pustules) occur, and although the disease involves the sebaceous areas, it often extends onto the scalp and arms. The mechanism is unknown, but may be similar to the pathogenesis of EGF-R inhibitor–induced folliculocentric lesions (see earlier in this article). The management of these patients is empiric, with agents such as those described for the EGF-R inhibitors.

In the larger paper, Mahé and colleagues [28] noted that 99% of the patients treated with sirolimus had one or more cutaneous adverse events, which included 20 of 95 patients who developed serious adverse reactions. Six of their patients discontinued therapy with sirolimus because of skin toxicity. Other than acne-like lesions, their patients had scalp folliculitis (26%), hidradenitis supprativa-like disease (12%), aphthous ulceration (60%), chronic gingivitis (20%), fissures of the lips (11%), and paronychia (16%). In addition, many of their patients experienced chronic edema that often lasted for more than 1 month and was nonresponsive to diuretic therapy. This latter adverse reaction occurred in 55% of their patients and in my view is not a cutaneous adverse reaction. Even eliminating this type of reaction, one is left with a high percentage of patients with skin toxicity. In addition, to the above-mentioned adverse reactions, these authors also observed a fairly large number of infections and malignancies within their patient population. These are also not traditionally considered to be adverse cutaneous reactions and it is believed by the author that they are not specific to this agent. The serious adverse events mentioned above included some patients with infections and when the data were examined closely, the reason for discontinuation of the sirolimus was usually because of some accompanying systemic toxicity and not solely because of a cutaneous adverse reaction. However, when sirolimus was discontinued, the cutaneous reactions halted or resolved.

Drug-induced lupus erythematosus

In 1985, Reed and colleagues [29] published the first case series of subacute cutaneous lupus erythematosus (SCLE) that was linked to the administration of a drug. In their report, the onset of the cutaneous eruption occurred during the administration of hydrochlorothiazide and resolved with its discontinuation. In addition, one of their patients had a second administration of hydrochlorothiazide that was followed by a reappearance of the eruption, which then cleared again with discontinuation of the offending drug. Their patients were anti-Ro (SS-A) positive, and in one of the three patients who was subsequently tested, the antibody disappeared.

Although there are multiple individual reports of drugs that have been associated with cutaneous LE, the largest series recently reported is that of Srivastava and colleagues [30]. They found that 15 of 70 patients with Ro (SS-A)–positive cutaneous lupus were associated with a recently administered drug (within the preceding 6 months). There are several issues that were raised by this paper. First, is the frequency outside of a tertiary center higher or lower than that observed in their report? Second, is the presence of the Ro (SS-A) antibody necessary for confirmation of the diagnosis of drug-induced LE? Third, are there other subsets of cutaneous LE that can be induced or exacerbated by drugs? Fourth, is it necessary to rechallenge patients to confirm a diagnosis of drug-induced SCLE? Fifth, how long an interval from initiation of a drug to the appearance of the eruption is acceptable? Sixth, what is the mechanism of induction of lesions; is the appearance of the skin lesions in these patients merely a reflection of the development of a photosensitive eruption in a patient with underlying SCLE or is this occurrence attributable to induction of antibodies that are pathogenetically involved in the production of the lesions? Last, since many of the patients with drug-induced disease continue to have cutaneous LE following the "induction" by the drug, what is the exact role of the drug—an initiator of disease or the awakening of an underlying disorder?

It is impossible to know what the true frequency of drug-induced SCLE is in the general community, but within our practice at the University of Louisville, it appears that roughly 10% of newly diagnosed patients with SCLE have a drug that is implicated. The diagnosis of SCLE is not dependent upon the identification of the Ro (SS-A) antibody; rather, it is a clinical diagnosis that is confirmed histopathologically. Therefore there may be many more patients with SCLE who were seen at this medical center. Their inclusion would then result in a lowering of the percentage of patients with SCLE who are linked to drug administration and would then be more reflective of the experience that we observed. What is needed is an examination of patients seen in a nonreferral setting that might reflect what is the true frequency in this environment.

The authors of this paper chose to include any patient with cutaneous LE who was diagnosed within 6 months of the administration of a "new" drug. Most drug eruptions occur within a short period of the administration of the drug and resolve relatively rapidly upon discontinuation of the drug. However, there are reports of minocycline-induced SLE that occur after long periods of administration of the drug, but these do resolve rapidly upon discontinuation of the minocycline [31]. The eruption began between 4 and 20 weeks after the offending drug was begun and resolved, generally with minimal intervention, between 6 and 12 weeks after discontinuation of the suspect drug. In this instance it seems reasonable to conclude that the drug was involved in the induction of the cutaneous disease because it might take a combination of the drug and light; furthermore, there might not be adequate amounts of light at the time that therapy with the drug is initiated.

Most of the patients in this report developed a photosensitive erythema, rather than classic annular or papulosquamous lesions of SCLE. Many of the drugs that are reported to be involved in this report are known to be photosensitizing agents and therefore one might wonder if the drug reaction reported herein is merely a phototoxic drug reaction in a patient who happens to possess Ro (SS-A) antibodies. This is less likely because of the observation that all of the patients had histopathology and immunofluorescence changes that were compatible with cutaneous LE. Another consideration for many of the patients with annular lesions of SCLE that have been previously reported is whether the occurrence is actually an erythema multiforme–like eruption in an Ro (SS-A)–positive patient. In this instance, the histology might also be represented by an interface dermatitis. This issue is not a factor in the current report.

Srivastava and colleagues [30] have also added two new classes to the already expanding list of drugs that are associated with drug-induced SCLE, as well as note a unique diagnostic problem. They reported on the first patients attributable to "statins" (lipid-lowering agents) and to interferon-alpha. The diagnostic problem that occurred involved the two patients in whom a "statin" was presumed to be the cause of the disease, as these patients also had an elevated creatine kinase and were weak. However, through careful evaluation, it became evident that these patients actually had two separate drug reactions, namely drug-induced myopathy and cutaneous lupus erythematosus. Therefore, the patients in whom "statins" have been linked to dermatomyositis-like disease should be reexamined for the possibility that they actually have SCLE. The authors of this report make a point to note that these two patients were Jo-1 negative. However, Jo-1 is not frequently present in dermatomyositis, and, therefore, its absence is not helpful in excluding a diagnosis of dermatomyositis. The basis of the diagnosis of drug-induced dermatomyositis should be the presence of clinically characteristic skin lesions, not a photosensitive eruption only.

They also identified two patients in whom the disease was attributable to a biologic agent—interferon-alpha in one and interferon-beta in another. Recent reports have documented the appearance of SCLE or SLE from etanercept, adalimumab, and infliximab. In a recent report, we noted that bupropion was the cause of SCLE [32]. Other drugs have subsequently been associated with the development of cutaneous LE (Box 1) [33–35].

Whether the appearance of the skin lesions in these patients is a reflection of the development of a photosensitive eruption in a patient with underlying SCLE or is attributable to the induction of Ro (SS-A) antibodies is not known. However, the observation by Srivastava and colleagues that the antibody titers dropped in most, and became undetectable in at least three patients, suggests that the drugs may induce antibodies that might be involved in the pathogenesis of the disease. However, there are multiple reports in which clinical and serologic disease continue following drug withdrawal. In these instances, the disease may be awakened by the drug and, once

Box 1. Drugs implicated in the development of cutaneous lupus erythematosus

Anti-hypertensive agents
  Thiazides diuretics
  Calcium channel blockers
  Angiotensin-converting enzyme
    inhibitors
  Beta blockers

Gastric acid–blocking agents
Nonsteroidal anti-inflammatory drugs
"Statins" (HMG CoA-reductase
  inhibitors)
Antifungals
  Griseofulovin
  Terbinafine

Antihistamines—cinnarazine
Anticonvulsants—phenytoin
Sulfonylureas
Chemotherapy—taxotere, tamoxifen
Miscellaneous—bupropion,
  TNF-antagonists, interferon-α and
  interferon-β, leflunomide, inhaled
  tiotropium

awakened, may continue. Further studies of prospectively identified patients might help us to elucidate the mechanism of this phenomenon.

What conclusions should be drawn from these and other observations of drug-induced SCLE? First, when making a diagnosis of SCLE, the practitioner must examine the drugs that the patient is taking to evaluate the possibility that a drug has caused or exacerbated the disease. Second, patients with "naturally" occurring SCLE should be advised about the risk of drugs that might exacerbate their disease. However, it should be stressed that it is not known what percentage of SCLE patients will experience an exacerbation of their disease with the appropriate use of anti-hypertensive agents including thiazides, ACE inhibitors, or calcium channel blockers. Therefore, when they are the best choice for the patient, they should be prescribed. Finally, the exacerbation of SCLE skin lesions caused by a drug, while distressing to the patient and physician, is not life-threatening and is usually treatable with drug discontinuation and standard forms of therapy used for LE.

Hand-foot syndrome

The hand-foot syndrome is characterized by painful acral eruption that consists of severe erythema with occasional bullae and erosions. It tends to be associated with cancer chemotherapy. Doxorubicin has been the most frequent agent associated with this process, but other agents have also been described. Two recent reports are worthy of mention. First, this reaction has been described following 3 months of therapy with fluvoxamine, a selective serotonin reuptake inhibitor used for depression [36]. Second, Chung and colleagues [37] reported a patient with clinical lesions of the hand-foot syndrome whose biopsy revealed a small-vessel vasculitis.

Summary

Many new drugs are entering the marketplace and although some cutaneous reactions might be noted in the preclinical evaluation, some of the reactions, particularly those that are rare, will not be noted until the drugs enter widespread use. In addition, distinctive reactions may occur, as is the case with epidermal growth factor–receptor inhibitors. Careful observation and evaluation might result in a better understanding of "naturally" occurring skin disease.

References

[1] Suntharalingam G, Perry MR, Ward S, et al. Cytokine storm in a phase 1 trial of the anti-CD28 monoclonal antibody TGN1412. N Engl J Med 2006;355: 1018–28.

[2] Drazen JM. Volunteers at risk. N Engl J Med 2006; 355:1060–1.

[3] Burgin S. New drugs, new rashes: update on cutaneous drug reactions. Adv Dermatol 2005;21:279–302.

[4] Perez-Soler R, Delord JP, Halpern A, et al. HER1/EGFR inhibitor-associated rash: future directions for management and investigation outcomes from the HER1/EGFR inhibitor rash management forum. Oncologist 2005;10:345–56.

[5] Perez-Soler R, Saltz L. Cutaneous adverse effects with HER1/EGFR-targeted agents: is there a silver lining? J Clin Oncol 2005;23:5235–46.

[6] Agero ALC, Dusza SW, Benvenuto-Andrade C, et al. Dermatologic side effects associated with the epidermal growth factor receptor inhibitors. J Am Acad Dermatol 2006;55:657–70.

[7] Seiverling EV, Fernandez EM, Adams D. Epidermal growth factor receptor (EGFR) inhibitor associated skin eruption. J Drugs Dermatol 2006;5:368–9.

[8] Laffitte E, Saurat J-H. Kinase inhibitor-induced pustules. Dermatology 2005;211:305–6.

[9] Roé E, Muret MPG, Marcuello E, et al. Description and management of cutaneous side effects during cetuximab or erlotinib treatments: a prospective study of 30 patients. J Am Acad Dermatol 2006; 55:429–37.

[10] Brazzelli V, Prestinari F, Roveda E, et al. Pityriasis rosea-like eruption during treatment with imatinib mesylate: description of 3 cases. J Am Acad Dermatol 2005;53(5 Suppl 1):S240–3.

[11] Dalmau J, Peramiquel L, Puig L, et al. Imatinib-associated lichenoid eruption: acitretin treatment allows maintained antineoplastic effect. Br J Dermatol 2006;154:1213–6.

[12] Ayirookuzhi SJ, Ma L, Ramshesh P, et al. Imatinib-induced sweet syndrome in a patient with chronic myeloid leukemia. Arch Dermatol 2005;141:368–70.

[13] Assouline S, Laneuville P, Gambacorti-Passerini C. Panniculitis during dasatinib therapy for chronic myelogenous leukemia. N Engl J Med 2006;354:2623–4.

[14] Thielen AM, Kuenzli S, Saurat J-H. Cutaneous adverse events of biological therapy for psoriasis: review of the literature. Dermatology 2005;211:209–17.

[15] Kary S, Worm M, Audring H, et al. New onset or exacerbation of psoriatic skin lesions in patients with definite rheumatoid arthritis receiving tumour necrosis factor alpha antagonists. Ann Rheum Dis 2006;65:405–7.

[16] de Gannes GC, Ghoreishi M, Pope J, et al. Psoriasis and pustular dermatitis triggered by tumor necrosis factor-α inhibitors in patients with rheumatologic conditions. Arch Dermatol, in press.

[17] Urbani R, Van Voorhees AS. Onset of psoriasis during treatment with tumor necrosis factor-alpha antagonists: three cases. Arch Dermatol, in press.

[18] Pirard D, Arco D, Debrouckere V, et al. Anti-tumor necrosis factor alpha-induced psoriasiform eruptions: three further cases and current overview. Dermatology 2006;213:182–6.

[19] Fiorentino DF. The Yin and Yang of TNF-α inhibition. Arch Dermatol, in press.

[20] Bleumink GS, ter Borg EJ, Ramselaar CG, et al. Etanercept-induced subacute cutaneous lupus erythematosus. Rheumatology 2001;40:1317–9.

[21] Fautrel B, Foltz V, Frances C, et al. Regression of subacute cutaneous lupus erythematosus in a patient with rheumatoid arthritis treated with a biologic tumor necrosis factor alpha-blocking agent: comment on the article by Pisetsky and the letter from Aringer et al. Arthritis Rheum 2002;46(5):1408–9.

[22] Norman R, Greenberg RG, Jackson JM. Case reports of etanercept in inflammatory dermatoses. J Am Acad Dermatol 2006;54(3 Suppl 2):S139–42.

[23] Winfield H, Lain E, Horn T, et al. Eosinophilic cellulitislike reaction to subcutaneous etanercept injection. Arch Dermatol 2006;142:218–20.

[24] Boura P, Sarantopoulos A, Lefaki I, et al. Eosinophilic cellutlitis (Well's syndrome) as a cutaneous reaction to the administration of adalimumab. Ann Rheum Dis 2006;65:839–40.

[25] Antiga E, Melani L, Cardinali C, et al. A case of lichenoid drug eruption associated with sildenafil citrates. J Dermatol 2005;32:972–5.

[26] Al-Shouli S, Abouchala N, Bogusz MJ, et al. Toxic epidermal necrolysis associated with high intake of sildenafil and its response to infliximab. Acta Derm Venereol 2006;85:534–5.

[27] Mahé E, Morelon E, Lechaton S, et al. Acne in recipients of renal transplantation treated with sirolimus: clinical, microbiologic, histologic, therapeutic, and pathogenic aspects. J Am Acad Dermatol 2006;55:139–42.

[28] Mahé E, Morelon E, Lechaton S, et al. Cutaneous adverse events in renal transplant recipients receiving sirolimus-based therapy. Transplantation 2005;79:476–82.

[29] Reed BR, Huff JC, Jones SK, et al. Subacute cutaneous lupus erythematosus associated with hydrochlorothiazide therapy. Ann Intern Med 1985;103(1):49–51.

[30] Srivastava M, Rencic A, Diglio G, et al. Drug-induced, Ro/SSA-positive cutaneous lupus erythematosus. Arch Dermatol 2003;139:45–9.

[31] Porter D, Harrison A. Minocycline-induced lupus: a case series. N Z Med J 2003;116(1171):U384.

[32] Cassis TB, Callen JP. Bupropion-induced subacute cutaneous lupus erythematosus. Australas J Dermatol 2005;46:266–9.

[33] Farhi D, Viguier M, Cosnes A, et al. Terbinafine-induced subacute cutaneous lupus erythematosus. Dermatology 2006;212:59–65.

[34] Rothfield N, Sontheimer RD, Bernstein M. Lupus erythematosus: systemic and cutaneous manifestations. Clin Dermatol 2006;24:348–62.

[35] Callen JP. How frequently are drugs associated with the development or exacerbation of subacute cutaneous lupus? Arch Dermatol 2003;139(1):89–90.

[36] Ke C-L, Chen C-C, Lin C-T, et al. Fluvoxamine-induced bullous eruption mimicking hand-foot syndrome and intertrigo-like eruption: rare cutaneous presentations and elusive pathogenesis. J Am Acad Dermatol 2006;55:355–6.

[37] Chung NM, Guiterrez M, Turner ML. Leukocytoclastic vasculitis masquerading as hand foot syndrome in a patient on Bay 43-9006. Arch Dermatol 2006;142:1510–1.

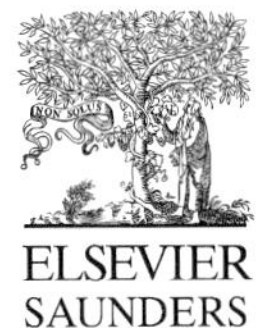

Dermatol Clin 25 (2007) 263–270

Index

Note: Page numbers of article titles are in **boldface** type.

A

Abacavir
and hypersensitivity syndrome, 248

Acitretin
dosage of, 191
and hair loss, 228
and skin cancer, 186, 188–189

Acne
and adrenal tumor, 141
and antibiotic resistance, 127–130
and congenital adrenal hyperplasia, 141
and dihydrotestosterone, 140–141
pharmacologic therapy for, 137–144
and retinoids, 151, 187
and tetracyclines, 134

Acne therapy
and oral contraceptives, 143–144

Adalimumab
and psoriasis, 209–210

Adult female acne, 143

Advances in topical and systemic antifungals,
165–183

Agranulocytosis
and hepatotoxicity, 199, 201–203

Alefacept
and psoriasis, 210–211

Allopurinol
and hypersensitivity syndrome, 247–248

Allylamines
and treatment of fungal infections, 176–177

Amphotericin B
and treatment of fungal infections, 167

Anagen effluvium, 223, 230

Androgen receptor blockers, 142–143

Anti-inflammatory activity of tetracyclines,
133–135

Anti-T-cell agents
and psoriasis, 210–211

Antibiotic cross-resistance, 130–131

Antibiotic resistance, 127–131
and acne, 127–130
and impact on commensal and transient
flora, 128–130
and mechanisms among bacteria, 129
patterns of, 130
and skin and soft tissue infections, 130
and tetracyclines, 127–130

Anticoagulants
and hair loss, 223

Anticonvulsants
and hypersensitivity syndrome, 246–247

Antidepressants
and hair loss, 227

Antiestrogens
and hair loss, 226

Antifungal agents, 165–180
and pharmacokinetic interactions, 170

Antimalarial agents
and hepatotoxicity, 201

Antineoplastic agents
and hair loss, 223–224

Antiretroviral drugs
and hair loss, 224

Anxiolytics
and hair loss, 227

Aplastic anemia
and hepatotoxicity, 199

Aromatase inhibitors
and hair loss, 226
Aspergillus infections
and caspofungin, 178–179
and micafungin, 179–180
and voriconazole, 173–174

Econazole
    and treatment of fungal infections, 168

Efalizumab
    and hepatotoxicity, 201
    and psoriasis, 210

Epidermal growth factor receptor inhibitors
    causing skin eruptions, 255–256
    Epidermophyton infections
    and griseofulvin, 175

Esterified estrogens-methyltestosterone
    replacement therapy
    and hair loss, 226

Etanercept
    and psoriasis, 207–209

Exanthematous pustulosis, 249

Extracorporeal membrane oxygenation
    and hair loss, 227

F

Fluconazole
    and treatment of fungal infections, 169

Fluoroscopy
    and hair loss, 227

Flutamide
    and sebaceous gland activity, 142–143

Fungal infections, 165–180

G

Gonadotropine-releasing hormone agonists
    and hair loss, 224

Granulomatous diseases
    and tetracyclines, 134

Griseofulvin
    and treatment of fungal infections, 175

H

Hair curling
    drug-induced, 224

Hair darkening
    drug-induced, 224

Hair graying
    drug-induced, 224

Hair growth
    excessive, 228–230

Hair loss
    and anticoagulants, 223
    and antidepressants, 227
    and antiestrogens, 226
    and antineoplastic agents, 223–224
    and antiretroviral drugs, 224
    and anxiolytics, 227
    and aromatase inhibitors, 226
    and busulphan, 228
    and chemotherapy, 223–224, 226
    diagnosis of, 229–230
    and dopaminergic therapy, 227
    drug-induced, 223–230
    and esterified estrogens-methyltestosterone
        replacement therapy, 226
    and extracorporeal membrane oxygenation,
        227
    and fluoroscopy, 227
    and gonadotropine-releasing hormone
        agonists, 224
    and interferons, 227
    and lichen planopilaris, 228
    management of, 229–230
    and minoxidil, 227
    and mood stabilizers, 227
    and oral contraceptives, 224
    permanent, 228
    and progestin-releasing implants, 224
    and psychotropic drugs, 227
    and radiation, 228
    and reninol, 227–228
    reversible, 223–228

Hair straightening
    drug-induced, 224

Hand-foot syndrome
    drug-induced, 260

Hemolysis
    and hepatotoxicity, 203

Hepatocellular toxicity monitoring, 198

Hepatotoxicity
    and agranulocytosis, 199, 201–203
    and antimalarial agents, 201
    and aplastic anemia, 199
    and azathioprine, 200
    and chlorambucil, 201
    classifications systems for, 196
    and colchicine, 201
    and cyclophosphamide, 201
    and dapsone, 200
    and differential diagnosis, 197
    and drug discontinuation, 201–202
    and drug hypersensitivity, 198